D1435346

Genius Breaks:
Optimize Your Workday
Performance and Well-Being

By Dr. Suzie Carmack

DEDICATION

Cynthia Marie Carmack
and
Patrick Earl Carmack

.

CONTENTS

Acknowledgments   i

1   Why You're a Genius and You Need to Take a Genius Break   9

2   How I Began This Journey In My Basement (and Became a Pioneer in the Fight Against Sitting Disease by Accident)   22

3   The ABCE Formula: How You Can Design Your Own Genius Break in 4 Easy Steps   44

4   The Genius Break 2/4/6/8/10 Movement Checklist: How To Move More Through Your Workday   63

5   Centering Self-Talk Themes: The Chakras of Communication   93

6   My Go-To Genius Break Practice For Extremely Busy People on Extremely Busy Days   108

7   The Geek Part If You Care: A White Paper on Sitting Disease (Sedentarism)   114

8   The Woo-Woo Part If You Care: A Very Brief Intro To Why Yoga Isn't About Being A Pretzel   128

Dr. Suzie Carmack, PhD, MFA, MEd, ERYT

You should consult your physician before engaging in this or any other physical activity program.

Avoid any movement that is painful or uncomfortable for you. Listen to your body's needs, and stay true to your self.

Disclaimer:
The activities and movements offered in this book are provided with an educational purpose only – and should not be misconstrued in any way as medical advice. If you choose to attempt the movements suggested in this book or in any of its related training programs, videos or materials, you accept any and all risks related to your participation, and release the author and her affiliates of any and all legal claims or judgments related to any discomfort or harm that may directly or indirectly ensue from your participation.

ACKNOWLEDGMENTS

Thanks to Grace Lever, for inspiring me to finally realize that one of my genius zones is helping others to take Genius Breaks – so that they can optimize their genius.

Thanks to my mentors, colleagues and students at George Mason University. Very special thanks to GMU's Dr. Gary Kreps, my doctoral advisor and mentor, who encouraged me to keep up the good fight against a chronic disease called sitting – before the world knew it was a problem.

Special thanks to Dr. Alfonso Contreras and the Pan American / World Health Organization for the opportunity to raise awareness about the workplace benefits of movement and mindfulness from 2013 - 2015. Special thanks to my movement and teachers over the past 50 years, especially Jodi Welch, Donna Grove, Renee Keil, Shane O'Hara, Linda Caldwell, Robert Ivey, Kathy Harty Gray, Michelle Larsson, Kevin Bowen, Lisa Johnson, Neva Ingalls, and so many other gifted souls from my yoga, Pilates, Laban/Bartenieff and modern dance training paths. When I move I hear you, and when I teach I share you.

Special thanks to four colleagues who are geniuses as well as dear friends: Dr. Suzanne Kennedy of the University of North Carolina; Dr. Denise Scannell of the MITRE corporation; Dr. Joshua Rosenberger of Pennsylvania State University and Alexis Rose of Keegan Theatre. Each of you has inspired me to never give up on my quirky perspective of scholarship and the world, and for that I will always be grateful.

And my deepest thanks to my beloved fiancée Bob and my amazing children Chris, Brandon and Sophia. I love you more than words can say.

1 Why You're a Genius and You (May) Need To Take A Genius Break

You are a genius.

Whether or not your I.Q. makes you an actual genius doesn't really matter.

You are a genius.

You have some type of genius skill – something that you are really good at, and you want to continue performing that skill as best as you can.

Like any genius, you like solving problems creatively. But you know that if you are not feeling well or are somehow off of you're A-game your work will suffer and you'll let your team down.

And, like any genius, you sometimes have a hard

time pulling away from the problem you are facing long enough to reboot yourself in ways that you know that you should. You feel torn between the idea of leaving the problem that you have become so attached to, and what you know to be true – that when you take a break to take care of yourself, you come back to whatever it is you were dealing with and whoever it is you are working with from a place that is more creative and less cranky.

Sound familiar?

As a geek (um, genius) who studies work/life balance in high consequence fields, I am personally fascinated (um, obsessed) with this dichotomy. We get so pulled into our work as geniuses, that at some point we over do it – and compromise the very work we are doing in the first place.

That's why I wrote this book.

Because, I bet you need a break.

A good one.

I invite you to take a break with me, with a special kind of break I call "Genius Breaks."

What's a Genius Break?

A Genius Break is a particular kind of break-taking – one that focuses on your performance optimization and personal well-being. Instead of being driven by your body's basic biological needs (like going to the bathroom or getting a snack), it's a specific type of break that you take to optimize your workday performance as well as your overall experience of work/life balance and well-being.

Genius Breaks help you to accomplish these professional and personal performance goals by combining movement, mindfulness and communication techniques into one simple and efficient practice that can be performed in as little as 2 minutes. Genius Breaks are designed to empower you to release mental, physical and emotional tensions in order to reboot your stamina, recharge your resilience, and reclaim your well-being.

So now you may be wondering, why do I need a break, let alone a Genius Break?

Well, if you're like me and you love what you do and/or you work in a high stakes field, you probably have a hard time taking breaks and pulling yourself a way from the genius work that you are doing. I conceptualize this dichotomy in my mind as a type of

genius overtraining. In athletics, overtraining is a particular syndrome that athletes can face if they push themselves "too much, too fast, or too soon" towards their performance goals. The sneaky and hard-to-detect syndrome can cause fatigue, anxiety, poor performance and an overall feeling of ill-being. Ironically, it is the athlete's commitment to excelling that both causes the problem and becomes the barrier to the athlete's success; they push themselves so hard that they go past their optimal training zone and end up compromising both their performance and their well-being. They overwhelm themselves by overdoing it.

In professional workplaces, I find many hard-driving and high-performing leaders and workers (geniuses like you) do the same thing, often having no idea that they are doing it. They are so committed to doing a good job and to excelling, that they push themselves past their own optimization point and end up jeopardizing both their performance quality and their personal well-being. They too overwhelm themselves by overdoing it.

This is one reason why lifeguards, police officers,

healthcare clinicians, air traffic controllers and pilots, have breaks that are professionally mandated. Unlike the rest of us who can choose whether or not we take breaks, workers in those fields don't get a choice -- they have to take breaks. It doesn't matter whether or not its easy for them to pull themselves away from the high consequence and high-demand work that they are doing, they have to take a break. Period.

Break-taking helps these workers to maintain the focus, vigilance and stamina they need to solve problems, prevent mistakes, and even save lives. Over the course of these workers' careers, break-taking can also help them to buffer the effects of burnout and compassion fatigue – which in turn can help to maintain their workplace and team engagement and personal job satisfaction.

I call out this example to you because I think all of us can learn from the example set by these workers in these and other high consequence fields.

Whether or not you are a worker or leader in these fields, and whether or not you have to take breaks because of a professional mandate, I ask you to consider that we can all make it our personal policy to take breaks during our workday or school day – in order to optimize both our workplace performance and our personal well-being.

So yes.

Go to the bathroom.

Go and get a (healthy) snack.

Go and walk the building (if you can safely).

Although these are not Genius Breaks, they are all standard forms of taking a break during your workday. And yes, I recommend that if you aren't taking these types of breaks on a regular basis that you start doing so immediately. For those of you who aren't working in high-paced fields, this might seem absurd that I am saying this. But for those of you who are working in a high-paced field, I know you are smiling because you know how difficult it can sometimes be to even consider doing any one of these activities during a day that has a jam-packed agenda – let alone all of them.

In addition to taking these very basic (bio) breaks, and honoring your very basic physiologic needs as a human, I also recommend that you take a Genius Break so that you really can optimize your workday performance and personal well-being.

Clearly, starting a Genius Break practice in your workplace (either on your own or with your team) will ask you to change the way you think about and perform the work that you do. The good news is that Genius Breaks have the potential to benefit your workplace performance as well as your personal well-being.

From a workplace optimization perspective, you might think of Genius Breaks as an "optimizing agent" for your performance effectiveness. Genius Breaks have the potential to benefit and improve your physical stamina (body), mental prowess (mind), and emotional resilience (heart). Not only is the act of taking a mindful movement break (or, Genius Break) good for your overall well-being for this "time out benefit," recent science has also demonstrated ways that mindfulness practices and movement practices can improve the functions of your body (vitality, stamina and energy level), your mind (cognition) and your heart (coping ability). Genius Breaks therefore have a potential "triple benefit" for your workday performance effectiveness, because you are experiencing all three benefits simultaneously. You are essentially improving your mind/body/heart operating system – enabling it to perform your work and to adapt to unforeseen stressors more efficiently.

Second, Genius Breaks are designed to improve your workplace performance by saving you time. They are actually themselves a form of "genius" in the sense that you don't have to take separate time out of your busy day to practice movement techniques and mindfulness techniques separately. Instead, these practices can be combined efficiently into one Genius Break that you can perform in as little as two minutes.

In addition to helping you to optimize your workday performance effectiveness and efficiency, Genius Breaks can also help you to improve your personal work/life balance and well-being. It is not surprising that workers who push themselves to meet high performance demands -- even when they love what they do – can easily fall prey to both burnout and compassion fatigue. These conditions not only threaten workplace performance safety, they also compromise personal well-being and the experience of work/life balance and vitality.

This book is therefore dedicated to helping you to optimize your workday performance (effectiveness and efficiency) and your personal well-being, by teaching you how you can design and perform your own Genius Breaks. This book also provides you with important contexts that will be helpful to you as you make and sustain your commitment to performing these Genius Breaks during your workday, and to (hopefully) sharing them with your colleagues and team.

In chapter 2, you'll learn the history behind Genius Breaks -- my personal story of how I began fighting sitting disease in 2007, and became a pioneer in the fight against sitting disease in my basement studio by accident. This chapter will teach you that I too have to work at maintaining my commitment to walking this walk – even as I continue to encourage other individuals and organizations around the world to do the same thing.

In chapter 3, you'll learn four easy steps to designing your own Genius Break – anytime and anywhere, including during your workday. This 4-step framework is the same one that I used to use to teach teachers and trainers how to create sessions for their clients. You'll go behind-the-scenes to learn the same framework (formula) so that you can design your own genius breaks in 4 easy-to-remember steps.

Then in chapter 4, you'll learn how to ensure that the movement portion of your Genius Break moves each of your joints appropriately and comprehensively, as I introduce you to the field of kinesiology using my "2/4/6/8/10" movement vitamin system. Think of this system as your own movement checklist – to ensure that your body has a minimal dose of daily movement in order to fight sitting disease and to sustain your overall health and well-being.

In chapter 5, you'll learn the mindfulness component of each Genius Break, through 8 themes which I call the chakras of communication. You'll discover how they can transform the intentionality (symbolism) of the movements you choose to do in each Genius Break – transforming each movement into a potential gesture (non-verbal form of communication) with yourself, your colleagues, and even the world at large. You'll also learn how you can use these 8 mindful communication themes to change your perception of your personal story, so that you can come back to your work (and your life) with a sense that you are writing the script of your workday experience no matter what may be happening around you and to you.

In addition to the history and context you'll find in chapter 2 and the "do-it-yourself details" you'll find in chapters 3 – 5, the remaining chapters of this book will share with you additional perspectives that may prove helpful to you as you start practicing Genius Breaks during your workday.

In chapter 6, I share my own "busy day" Genius Break practice which you are welcome to copy and follow. (I also have a video of this practice posted on my website at www.DrSuzieCarmack.com). In chapter 7, I share my research on the dangers of sitting-too-much and in chapter 8, I give you a very quick glimpse into yoga philosophy. Please keep in mind that although Genius Breaks do not look like any traditional "asana" yoga practice, they are inspired by the self-awareness and self-care benefits that come from a regular yoga practice -- as well as any other regular practice of Pilates or other forms of mindful movement.

But before we get to all of that and get you moving, I have one more appeal for you – especially if you happen to be a leader of a team.

Please don't perform these Genius Breaks alone. Please encourage your team to join you.

Why?

We humans are like birds. We aren't quite sure what to do when one person flies off, away from the flock to do their own thing. But if a few people follow that strange outlier (and engage in a new behavior) suddenly the whole flock (team, family, group of friends) follows along too.

And that is why I ask you here to not just design and perform these Genius Breaks - but to also get anyone and everyone you know to perform them too. It's time that we all chose to be "that person…" who encourages people in meeting or a class session to pause long enough to move mindfully and reboot the mind, body and heart.

So let's do this.

When we know we need a Genius Break, but we

aren't sure if others around us will approve, let's not stay silent. And, let's certainly not sit still.

Instead, let's ask everyone around us to join us, so that we ourselves feel that we aren't alone.

Let's make sure our teams feel supported in this idea of Genius Break-taking so that workplace norms can change and that all of us feel supported in taking any type of break – bio breaks and Genius Breaks.

And together we can make it so that each of us are not only performing our work optimally and experiencing well-being – but that sitting disease is an extinct epidemic.

Let's take our evolution back to vertical.

Let's get started.

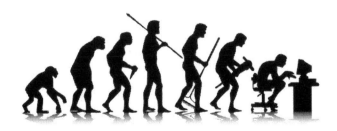

2 How I Began This Journey In My Basement (and Became a Pioneer in the Global Fight Against Sitting Disease by Accident)

If you're wondering why a yoga teacher like me became a pioneer in the global fight against sitting disease, and found herself delivering much of the material you'll find in this book to the World Health Organization through keynotes and workshops, this chapter is for you. If it really doesn't matter to you how or why that happened, and you want to find out how you can create your own Genius Breaks in as little as two minutes, then feel free to skip this chapter and move on to chapter three.

If you're still reading here and haven't jumped ahead, that means you're curious about my story and why I wrote this book. So, here we go.

It was 2007, and I lived with my family in Lorton, Virginia, a little suburb south of Washington, DC. I was fortunate to be one of those very lucky moms who worked about 25 – 30 hours per week around the needs of my children, who were aged 12, 11 and 6 years.

In my professional time, I was a kinesiologist (movement scientist), yoga therapist, and international yoga trainer – which meant that I worked with my own clients one-on-one, taught classes, and traveled throughout the U.S. (and sometimes abroad) to run certification weekends for yoga teachers. I also taught yoga and Pilates at the local community college, and danced in a professional modern dance company. In my civic time, I choreographed musicals for the local high school as a way to "give back" to our local community.

Today I lead a much different life, as a health communication scholar, strategist and speaker. I design interventions that study ways that mindfulness, movement and communication training can promote workplace compassion and engagement and prevent burnout and compassion fatigue in healthcare and other high consequence and high performance fields.

But I share this snapshot of my work and my life from 2007 with you here for an important reason. Although my Genius Breaks have been developed based on recent research establishing the importance of taking mindfulness and movement breaks for optimal workday performance, they were actually inspired by my prior work as a movement scientist and mindfulness coach in private practice from 2001 – 2011 and even my prior work as a fitness instructor from 1997 - 2001. As you'll learn in a moment, it was during that period of my work that I was inspired to start fighting a disease called sitting – completely by accident – long before the world knew about standing desks and treadmill desks.

What I didn't realize at the time, but can see so clearly now, is that by 2007 I was working with almost every developmental age in my private movement and mindfulness coaching practice. Now that I am a scholar and a strategist, I realize how lucky I was to essentially have the opportunity to do informal observational research and intervention development with each population (although I did not conceptualize it as such at the time).

As a free-lancer all that I wanted was to work at times that were convenient for my own work/life balance, and for my primary role as a mother of three. That drive to build my work around my availability (and not the other way around) led me to work with populations based on their availability – which is how I accidentally ended up working with so many different client age populations.

To explain further what I mean by different population and developmental age groups, and to give you a little more insight into how Genius Breaks were inspired, allow me to describe a typical workday at the time the idea for them started - in 2007.

In the early mornings, I worked with early birds and professionals (aged 40 – 72 years) in one:one movement training sessions. Many of these clients were my "seven and seven" clients – they often worked from 7 AM to 7 PM as devoted public servants in Washington, DC (i.e., government folks, military personnel, and anyone else committed to national advocacy). They would hire me to move them in some way (Pilates, yoga, or personal training) or to teach them how to manage the work-related stress that comes with working in high performance environments. I'd wrap up the movement portion of their session with a mindfulness theme or inspiring thought for the day, and send them on their way to go take on the world's business - literally.

For the rest of the morning, I got my own elementary school-aged children (aged 6 – 12 years) moving as I fed them and took them to their respective schools. Around lunchtime, I drove to the community college to teach Yoga and Pilates– which gave me the opportunity to work with traditional college students (aged 18 – 22 years) as well as non-traditional students (aged 23 – 67 years).

If it was a rehearsal day, I spent some of the afternoon working with high school-aged children (13 – 17 years) as the choreographer for the drama department. And, about one weekend per month I would travel to lead a certification training weekend, which meant working with teacher trainees (aged 17 years and up).

So as you can see, I was working one way or another with almost every possible developmental age

— unintentionally, and without even stopping to realize it.

Back then, all I knew was that as I got to know my clients and students, I was able to observe them as individuals, and to find preference trends amongst them. I learned what movement and mindfulness practices did and didn't work for each individual, and each group. Over time, I learned how to congratulate them when they achieved a milestone and how to console them when they fell short of their performance goals.

And above all, I learned to combine preparation with improvisation -- to go into each session with a checklist so that I was prepared, but to be ready for any and all possibilities to improvise off of it as necessary so that both the client/student and I could perform as well as possible. Their real-time needs and ever-changing capabilities taught me to always begin each session by being as present as possible, and to work my plan while making my plan work.

Suffice it to say that I had to stay mindful as I was teaching them how to mindfully move.

I share the fact that I was working with, adapting

to, and learning from each of these developmental age groups, because it provides an important background and context for what I'm about to share next.

In the Spring of 2007, I started to notice something happening in all of the settings I worked in, and with all of the age groups I was working with. A truth was emerging that gave me a funny feeling at the bottom of my stomach.

Everyone was moving less.

And…

[Here comes the scary part.]

As far as I could tell, no one else seemed concerned about it

[Gulp.]

Now you may think I'm being overly dramatic, but you have to realize that at the time, no one was talking about sitting disease, or other technology-induced stress factors in the workplace. We not only didn't have treadmill desks or wearables (like FitBits), we didn't know we even needed them. Both iPhone and Playstation 3 had just come out that year (2007) – and we didn't yet know what an iPad or other mid-sized devices were because they would not be invented for another three years.

So back then, in 2007, I wasn't sure if it was just my own passion for movement that was making me paranoid that my clients seemed to be sitting more – or if there was indeed a real problem on the horizon.

After about a year's time, it seemed that the problem wasn't going away and might actually be getting worse. All of the groups I worked with (in every age population I taught), continued to report that they were moving less and stressing more. I decided that I needed to validate what I was seeing – to see if I literally was not the only one with this point of view. I wanted to see if what I was seeing in my own limited circle of influence was true elsewhere – or if I needed to get help for my (potentially) paranoid belief.

So one day during an advanced certification weekend (where I was teaching a workshop with experienced instructors), I asked the teachers I was training if they too were noticing that their clients were moving less and stressing more, due to technology.

It overwhelmed me how fast they said…

"YES!"

The floodgates opened.

They started telling me story after story of how they were seeing their clients move less and stress more. They were seeing the same things I was seeing – in all age populations. Some of them were moms like me, and they told me how they saw the same thing happening with their own children too. They admitted that they also had not been sure if was "just them" or if there was a real problem going on.

We all kept nodding and smiling at each other. I was overcome with a dual-edged feeling. On the one hand I was relieved to know I wasn't alone in seeing the problem – while at the same time I had a deeper sense of fear in knowing that the risk was not just in my or their imagination.

In the space of one breath I had mixed emotions. On my exhale, I breathed a sigh of relief, comforted by the fact I wasn't paranoid after all. On the next inhale, I realized we were all breathing into an emerging problem that would change the way the world was living and working.

There was an uncomfortable moment in the

silence of my next breath or two.

And then the funniest, and perhaps most ironic moment happened.

Someone, in this room of movement teachers shared that they admitted that they too were moving less and sitting more. I chimed in immediately and said, "Me too." We all laughed at the irony, that we were movement teachers and we were moving less and sitting more. We then went back to the workshop's content, and literally moved on.

But later as I reflected on the day during my flight back home, I realized it really wasn't a laughing matter after all. It was the beginning of a shift – in me, and in the way I saw the world.

When I got back to my private practice the next week I knew that there was no way that I could ever stop the technology changes that were causing the problem in the first place, so I decided that I should at least do what I could for my own clients to help them to adapt and cope with the new demands that were coming with this new technology. I decided it was best to start with doing what I could for my seven-and-seven clients. I knew that of all of the age groups I was working with, they were moving the least and sitting the most.

So that week during my lesson prep for my weekly client sessions, I started experimenting with ways that I could practice yoga poses without completely leaving my desk. At first I played with bringing my yoga mat to my workstation, but soon I realized that most of my clients did not and would not have a mat anywhere near their desk. So I started experimenting with ways that I could move while seated in the chair and with using both the desk and the chair as fitness equipment.

As a Pilates instructor trained in apparatus-work, I knew how to creatively use non-traditional equipment to both support a rehabilitative client and to challenge an athletic client. So, I applied those skills to my own work station, and the idea for what we now know to be Genius Breaks was born (although I didn't call it that at the time).

Soon I was developing customized movement routines for each of my clients based on their physical abilities and what I knew about their work places. I then spent some time in each of their regular training sessions teaching them these routines, and told them that these routines were 'Homework' for them to practice between our sessions to accelerate our session-based work.

The first time I introduced this idea to one of my long-time clients, I expected her to be skeptical. She liked to work hard, in a no-frills and no-time-to-waste kind of way. I didn't think she'd want to spend the time in our regular session learning this desk-based routine.

Her reaction was surprisingly very positive. "I love this," she said. She liked the simplicity of the movements, even though they were not as rigorous or as demanding as her normal workout. I confirmed to her that she should think of this as mindful movement -- not exercise.

The session went well, and she caught onto the desk-based routine I had given her very quickly. But at the end of the session she said to me, "I'm not sure how everyone at the office is going to react to this."

I asked her if she had an office with a door on it, and she said yes. So I encouraged her to close her door and do the movements solo for now. She surprised me during our next session when she told me she had been brave enough to share the movements with her team and they had fun trying them as a "team-building activity."

And so that was how it all began in my basement movement studio – my personal crusade to get people moving more and sitting less, as well as my belief that bringing mindful movement into the workday is good for both leaders and their teams.

I continued to develop customized routines for my other corporate and personal training clients, and before I knew it I was teaching them to my high school and college students too. I was also bringing them to my children's schools as a classroom volunteer.

By 2010, bringing mindful movement to workplaces and schools had become a key part of my personal training business. I also began leading specialty certification workshops that taught other yoga and movement teachers how they could create and share these desk-chair routines with their clients in their communities. And, I was delivering lunch-and-learn workshops for both small and large (fortune 500) corporations, to help their organizations and their teams to move more and sit less. To quote a well-known song from the 1980's, one thing really did lead to another.

By 2011, I decided that it was time that I learned more about the art and science of promoting health behavior change – to learn the science behind what I had been doing intuitively. That decision soon led me to George Mason University, where I would earn a PhD in health communication from 2011-2014. My doctoral training there exposed me to some of the world's best scholars in health communication, and enabled me to take elective graduate-level courses in epidemiology and public health.

Over the course of those 3 years, I had the support I needed to research the problem of sitting too much, and to address it through health communication and health promotion.

Along the way, I learned research skills which led me to unearth a small but growing body of literature that had identified something called "sedentarism" (which we now know as sitting disease) as the fourth largest global health risk. I discovered that back in

2001, before I had noticed any changes in my own clients' and family's movement patterns, a scholar named Booth had called the problem "sedentary death syndrome," and that both his alarming term to describe the problem and his work never caught the full public health attention they deserved. I discovered that over 26 different health conditions were caused by or made worse by sitting too much and other forms of physical inactivity.

But the biggest discovery I made was actually not made in the classroom or during my research activities.

Over the course of those 3 years of intense study, my biggest revelation was that I had to sit a lot to learn how to fight the sitting problem.

Yep.

I spent a lot of time sitting while I was learning how to better fight the global epidemic of sitting disease.

I sat while I researched.

I sat while I wrote papers.

I sat while I drove to the university.

I sat in meetings with my advisors.

I sat while I attended 3-hour graduate classes.

Yes, you read that correctly.

I was sitting too much in order to fight the problem of sitting too much.

I had become my own subject.

I had become my own client.

So that is when it happened – my epiphany.

On the one hand, I felt deeply embarrassed that I was becoming part of the sitting problem – that I had become one of my own clients.

On the other hand, I felt enlightened to be able to get inside of my own protocol. Like a doctor that one day becomes a patient, and finally "gets" the patients' point of view in ways that were not previously possible, the tables had finally turned. I was my own client. I could finally see what I previously couldn't see from the outside looking in to my movement and mindfulness intervention. I saw what needed further refinement, and I experienced barriers to the solution that I would have not otherwise known.

Inspired by both this epiphany and my new-found perspective, I did two things.

First, I started practicing the same routines I had

spent so many years developing for my clients, for my students and had taught other instructors to share with their clients and students. This became especially important as I was spending less time teaching yoga and movement classes, and more time studying, researching and writing.

Second, I also revised my approach and shared it with trainers at a regional fitness training conference. I called it "The Movement Vitamin: Your Daily Dose of Kinesiology." That turned out to be a pivotal moment in my work, although I didn't realize it at the time.

At the end of the session, a woman came up to me and thanked me for the workshop, and I thanked her for attending. As I started to gather my things to leave, she mentioned that her name was Vicki Hallet, and that she was the fitness reporter from the *Washington Post*.

No one was more surprised than me – I had no idea that she was coming, and had not realized while I was presenting that I was doing so in front of the media.

She explained that she was attending the

conference for her own training and development, not as a reporter. But then she went on to tell me that she felt what I had shared in the workshop would be beneficial to her colleagues as well as her readers, and that she wanted to follow-up with me. She invited me to visit the *Post's* offices and to lead some of their team through a mini-class. And she wrote an article to share some of the ideas I had shared in my workshop.

When her article came out, she described her experience of the mindful movement break I had shared with her and her colleagues at the office of the *Post* as her "new office habit". No one was more surprised than me that the article was redistributed in 89 news outlets, and suddenly the world was talking about this idea of "working out at your work station" and "exercising at your desk."

I didn't really care about the 10 minutes of fame I personally experienced based on this worldwide coverage of my work. All I knew was that I was glad that people were finally hearing an important message – that they needed to start making an effort to sit and stress less and move more during their workday, for their own health, longevity, and quality of life. This is a message that I continue to try to share whenever I can today, and the key message of this book.

After the *Post* article came out in September 2012, I continued to juggle my PhD studies and research with the occasional workshop delivery. I also maintained my private practice with a few clients, and continued to refine my approach based on their feedback. By the end of 2012, I had also presented my research at major conferences, like the American Public Health Conference, and the National Academies of Practice.

And all the while the world continued to sit more because technology continued to evolve.

And all the while I continued to sit more because I too was evolving -- into a scholar.

But I kept practicing the mindful movement breaks in order to keep up with the growing demands of my work, as well as my personal life's demands. And, I kept tweaking them in my personal practice for my own needs.

Then in 2013, I got a call from a student who had seen one of my lectures at George Mason University in her graduate public health class. She invited me to come to the Pan American / World Health Organization (PAHO/WHO) where she also worked, and to teach their team my mindful movement "sitting disease intervention" as part of their international offices' wellness week.

I gladly accepted, thinking that I might be in some type of alternate universe, and that I would wake up any minute. For someone who was still in doctoral training in global and community health, and still learning best practices in health communication, the fact that PAHO/WHO was calling me to come in and give a keynote and lecture/demonstration that would be telecast to their offices throughout the Americas felt a little like I imagine being nominated for an Academy Award feels like for an actor.

I was honored to not only deliver the keynote n 2013, but to also be invited back to PAHO/WHO for two more years during their wellness weeks, and to keep working with them on ways to get people to move more and practice mindfulness during the workday. We produced some YouTube videos which teach people how to move and practice mindfulness in short mini-breaks or 'activity pauses' as they call them. My work with PAHO/WHO also opened another door for my work with the National Parks Service. I was honored to help them and the U.S. Surgeon General to launch their Park RX campaign in April of 2016. The now-national campaign encourages people to consider going outside (even during the workday) to be a "prescription" for their health and well-being.

So there you have it – that's my story of how I became a pioneer in the fight against sitting disease by accident, and how it all started in my basement studio.

But the best part of all for this story, is the epilogue.

As I write to you now, 10 years after I had that funny feeling in my stomach in 2007 I find it perhaps the biggest plot twist of all that I have literally become one of my seven-to-seven clients.

Today, I spend my weeks working as a scholar and strategist in the field of health communication, teaching at George Mason University and developing evidence-based interventions that promote work/life balance and prevent workplace burnout. I also speak consult and coach as my schedule permits.

I am able to keep this pace, and stay engaged in my work in these high performance contexts, because I continue to practice Genius Breaks as part of my daily commitment to self-care.

And that's why I decided that it was finally time to write this book and its accompanying online training program – exactly 20 years after I began my movement coaching career as a group fitness instructor and 10 years after I noticed that people were sitting too much every day.

Today, I see the same trend that bothered me so much in 2007 not being adequately addressed by treadmill desks, standing desks, and wearables. It is my hope that by sharing my work through this book that we all – myself included -- take the time to take better care of ourselves by moving more.

So now that you know my story a little better, let's get you started on the journey to designing your own Genius Breaks -- so that you can move more and sit less and optimize your workday performance and personal well-being.

3 THE ABCE FORMULA: HOW YOU CAN DESIGN YOUR OWN GENIUS BREAK IN 4 EASY STEPS

It's time now to take the first step in getting you started on designing your own Genius Breaks. Think of this formula – as your choreographic recipe for creating your own unique Genius Breaks.

A: Assess (Time, Tone and Self)

B: Breath and Bones (Move Using 2/4/6/8/10)

C: Centering Communication (Self-Talk Themes)

E: Experience (Engage, Embrace, Embody, Evaluate)

Let's now explore 4 easy and simple steps you can use to bring this formula to life – and to perform your own Genius Breaks at work, at school, and at home (or anywhere you need a Genius Break!)

Step 1: Assess (Time Tone and Self)

Time: Decide how long you will give yourself to take your Genius Break, and set a timer if you need one so that you can focus on the break (and not on the worry that you will miss an important deadline if you stop to perform it). Ideally, you should plan each Genius Break for at least 10 minutes but if your time is limited your body will benefit from a break that is as little as 2 minutes. (To learn more about how beneficial hormonal changes can occur when you stand and move into power poses for at least 2 minutes, please see the work of Amy Cuddy).

Space: Once the time is set, be sure that you assess and secure your space, and that you have ample room to move safely. Look around you in a 360-degree view, and make sure you do not have any people or things that would get in your way while you move, so that you can stay safe and secure. If others are joining you, make sure that they too are safe and secure.

Self: After you have set the time for your Genius

Break, turn off your computer, shut your door, or take some other action that tells the world this is your time – even if it is only for 2-10 wonderful minutes. This act, however small, sets the tone for the Genius Break and tells your mind, body and heart, that it is time to participate in, and receive the benefits from, your Genius Break.

Once you feel you can truly begin, close your eyes and reflect on where your mind, body and heart were before you decided to take this Genius Break. Imagine that each of them is personified as a member of a committee meeting. Ask them (your internal team) to each report in on what this moment "means" to each of them.

For example, your body may report, "This is an opportunity for me to change position; I've been sitting all day".

Your mind may report, "This is an opportunity for me to step back and reboot so that I can stay alert and focused on that project we are working on".

Your heart may report, "This is an opportunity for me to release my worries over what's not working, and to renew my commitment to what needs to happen."

Next, thank your body, mind and heart for these "reports," no matter how favorable or unfavorable they may be. Then, become your own "CEO" and decide how you want your mind body and heart to experience the Genius Break from this moment forward based on this assessment that you have just completed. Set the outcomes you wish to achieve for yourself in this Genius Break, and keep them in mind as you go through the remaining steps.

Then communicate these outcomes to each "committee member" (i.e., your mind body and heart). For example, you may tell your body that its desired outcome goal is to release tension and/or to feel more reenergized. You might tell the mind that its intended outcome goal is to feel more relaxed and/or more refreshed. You might tell the heart that its intended outcome goal is to feel released from worries and/or renewed in its commitment to engage with the workday's demands.

As you communicate these outcome goals to your mind, body and heart, let go of any worries that may creep up that the break will not be performed long enough or well enough. These performance fears are common and are just your "ego" talking, which always thinks that your performance is never enough. If you are performing well, it wants more of the same, and if you are not performing well it will tell you it wants something else. You are enough. And, no matter how much mastery you do or don't feel you have in them, each Genius Break itself is enough. Reassure yourself that even a small amount of break-taking is beneficial for your workday performance and personal well-being – because it is.

Step 2: Breath and Bones (Move in 2/4/6/8/10)

Once you have set your mental, physical, and/or emotional outcome goals for the session (in step 1) it is time to focus on the movement portion of the break with your "B's" – your bones and your breath.

Breath First, notice your breath. Allow yourself several cycles in which you lengthen your inhales and exhales. Take in more air than you normally do on your inhale, and let out more air than you normally do on your exhale. If this makes you feel uncomfortable in any way, choose to omit this type of conscious breathing, and go back to your normal pace and quality of breath. If possible, aim to breathe lower into your abdomen (and not high into your chest, as this type of breath is associated with a heightened (anxious) stress response).

If you are able to perform these cycles of bigger breaths comfortably, imagine that you are flushing your body of stale air – much like you would open a window to a stale room. This will help you to stay connected to your breath throughout your practice, and will help you to engage your core more effectively (since many of your deep, interior, core muscles are actually some of the same muscles you use for breathing well).

Next, take a moment to recognize your overall energy level in your mind, body and heart. If you feel sluggish, take a few extra breaths in which you breathe in longer than you breathe out. If you feel anxious, take a few breaths in which you breathe out longer than you breathe in. Then, take several cycles in which you breathe in an equal ratio (with your inhales of the same duration as your exhales).

As you prepare to move you want to try to sustain this commitment to conscious breath as much as you comfortably can. Conscious breathing can help you to clear your mind, and also to execute whatever movements you do in a more controlled way that more effectively engages your interior (core) musculature.

You can begin whatever movement patterns you choose to perform in this Genius Break by remembering that your inhales will help you to feel expansive, and your exhales will help you to feel controlled and grounded. So, if you aren't sure where, when and how to breathe when you are moving, it might help to remember that when you performing movements that open your body outward (bringing your arms and legs away from your midline), you might enjoy inhaling. When you are performing movements that close your body (bringing your arms and legs closer to your midline), you might enjoy exhaling. Feel free to adjust this as you feel comfortable, and to remember that when all else fails please don't stop breathing. ☺

Bones Whether you have 2 minutes, 10 minutes, 30 minutes or more, take the time to ensure that your body completes at least one set of 2/4/6/8/10 movements. If you don't know yet what I mean by this, be sure to check out chapter four, where I explain this "mindful movement vitamin" that I developed back in 2008.

You'll learn in that chapter that by choosing to engage your hinge joints (elbows and knees) in two directions, your spine in four directions, your hips in six directions and your shoulders in eight directions, that you will have essentially engaged all of your major muscle groups by moving all of your major joints in all three planes of motion. That is why I use my 2/4/6/8/10 system (movement vitamin) to make sure I myself have moved all of my joints on a given day, and that I have moved my clients or students in all directions during a session in ways that support symmetry and avoid under- or over-training a particular muscle group.

Once you learn the 2/4/6/8/10 system in chapter 4 (or online in one of my training videos), you'll find that its easy to make up your own routines, and to share them with others at your office. I only ask that you please make sure that you and whoever you are practicing with feels safe, and that you and they do not do anything that does not feel right for your mind or your body. Be sure that you are having fun while you move – because that is ultimately what makes or breaks whether or not you continue.

Step 3: Centering Communication Theme

After you have decided which movements you will be performing as part of your Genius Break (step 2), you can next choose to add a centering theme to your movement pattern (Step 3). In this way, your daily Genius Break becomes more than just a physical fitness exercise or movement routine. With the addition of a centering communication theme, your movement can not only serve this fitness purpose, but also transform into a communicative gesture.

By taking time to consider your movement as a form of communication, you can step back from your day's demands long enough to decide how you would like to rewrite your self-talk and perform your story – which will in turn help you to not only manage the day's stressful demands, but to exercise your resilience and coping capability.

In chapter 5 you will learn the specific 8 centering themes I recommend for your Genius

Breaks, which I also call the chakras of communication. Here you will learn how these 8 themes are grouped into three primary categories (Intrapersonal, Interpersonal and Intercultural), and how each of these communication themes is inspired by each of the eight energy centers that are known in Eastern medicine as the chakra system.

Under this mind-body medicine paradigm, the lower body is symbolic of our (intrapersonal) relationship with ourselves, our mid-body is symbolic of your (interpersonal) relationship with others, and our whole body is symbolic of our (intercultural) relationship with the world. If you are not familiar with mind-body medicine in general or the chakra system in particular, this concept may be difficult to grasp, and that's OK.

One way that may be helpful for you to understand how these centering communication themes (chakras of communication themes) can nevertheless work for you even if you find them confusing or a bit too 'woo woo' for your liking, is to consider that any movement can be thought of as a physical experience, as an emotional gesture of communication, or in the case of a Genius Break – as both. So, that means that whatever 2/4/6/8/10 movements you choose in step 2 can be used to reinforce any centering self-talk messages you want to send to yourself (and others).

Essentially, through your centering communication theme you can transform your movement into a moving mantra.

For example, you might be feeling as though you would like to build the self-confidence you need to feel like you are "standing on your own two feet" in your life. This idea could be reinforced during your Genius Break by taking time to literally stand on your own two feet, and to connect into the strength of your lower body. You could then repeat to yourself (either out-loud or within your own mind's eye) the phrase "I stand on my own" or "I am stomping out difficulty." This would be an example of an intrapersonal message being reinforced by the lower body's posture of standing or gesturing of stomping. Said another way, the non-verbal movement of standing and stomping reinforces the self-talk reaffirming phrase (mantra) – whether or not it is said aloud.

Another example of how movement can be considered a moving mantra, or self-talk expression, can be illustrated in the following example. Imagine you would like to stay fearless in an upcoming meeting – to not feel bullied into making a wrong decision. This idea could be reinforced by first picking a movement that occurs somewhere near or around the heart center, because from a mind-body paradigm perspective, it is our house of both fear and love.

Once you choose a movement that helps you to open your chest and to feel fearless and expansive in this center (for example, opening your arms wide like you are about to give a hug), you might add in the repetition of a self-talk phrase (mantra) that reinforces this concept. You might say to yourself in your mind's eye or out-loud, "I am opening up to new possibilities," while you literally open your arms for a hug. You might then close your eyes as you imagine your whole body feeling fearless, courageous, and expansive. This would be an example of an interpersonal message being reinforced by the mid-body's gesture. As with the first example of "standing on your own two feet," the non-verbal movement reinforces the self-talk phrase – whether or not it is said aloud.

As noted above, you'll learn more about these 8 chakras of communication, and how you can use them to center yourself through positive self-talk in chapter 5. There you will learn that these 8 centering self-talk themes (which I call the chakras of communication) are: respect (feet), gratitude (hips), commitment (belly), courage (heart), kindness (mouth and arms), insight (forehead), community (crown of head) and consciousness (whole body / beyond body). Each communication theme has a very specific reason for being related to a particular zone (chakra) of the body under the mind/body paradigm, but you can feel free to choose any theme to go with any type of movement – as long as it makes you feel empowered during your Genius Break ☺.

Step 4 (E): Experience: Engage, Embrace, Embody, Evaluate and Ending

Once you have chosen how to link your movement to one of these centering themes, you then simply experience the Genius Break itself. To optimize your experience of your Genius Break, think of this fourth and final step of experience as being a combination of four mini-steps: engagement, embrace, embodiment, and evaluation. Your ultimate goal is to combine these mini-steps in ways that help you to optimally experience both the movement and the centering theme you have chosen, in ways that are in alignment with the same outcome goals that you set in step 1.

Engage: Remember that when you begin to engage (perform) your Genius Break, that it is important to take an improvisational approach to doing so. Remind yourself that no matter how your practice actually goes, it really is ok. A Genius Break is an ultimate opportunity to engage with your self. Do your best to be "all-in" – by tuning out distractions, by not trying to multi-task, and by not talking yourself out of it before you even give yourself a chance to get started.

Embrace: As you fully engage in the performance of your Genius Break, it is also important for you to fully embrace yourself – flaws and all. You are practicing Genius Breaks, not trying to perfect them. Let go of any self-criticism or self-judgment you have of your own capabilities to plan, to move, to breathe, to self-talk -- and just have fun. (The act of doing so will also help you to practice the art of being less critical and more accepting throughout the rest of your workday – another added benefit for your workday experience and performance). This is one of the reasons that I created a system that you could make up your own movements in – rather than giving you a prescribed routine. Everyone has their own capabilities, preferences, strengths, and quirks. Have fun embracing all of these within yourself, and move through any self-doubt that gets in the way of your embrace of yourself.

Embody: Remember that your break is designed to help you to become more embodied during your workday – which more than likely asks you to live more in your head and less in your body and your heart. Take the time to acknowledge the needs of your mind (thoughts), your body and your heart (feelings) – as discussed in step 1. Then, do your best to both create and experience the Genius Break in ways that are consistent with the outcome goals you set at the top of your practice.

One way to embody your break is to close your eyes and ask anyone else you are practicing with to do the same. Then, try to get inside of the joy that connects your mind, body and heart when you move mindfully and without self-doubt or self-criticism. Remember that before you close your eyes to move, that you should first check the scene around you to be sure that you are safe to do so (see step 1) ☺.

Evaluation: Once your experience of the break is over, through this combination of engagement, self-embrace and embodiment, it is time to take a deep breath or two and to evaluate how you feel the Genius Break as compared to your outcome goals. Take the time to consider that no matter what your experience was for this Genius Break, that it was an opportunity for you to reboot yourself so that you can return to your workday refreshed and recharged, AND to learn about yourself in the process. Give yourself at least one "glow" (congratulate yourself for one positive experience in your Genius Break) and one "grow" (offer yourself one way you can do better the next time you perform a Genius Break).

Ending: Much like no one likes it when a meeting ends abruptly and everyone scatters without even saying good-bye, your mind, body and heart deserve the same courtesy of being thanked for their participation. This means that you should take time to thank yourself for your practice, and to prepare to transition into whatever is next in your workday.

In my yoga and movement instructor-training workshops, I over-emphasize this point because I find it to be an often-missed step for many instructors. They are so dedicated to building a strong class experience, that they either don't manage the timing of the class and/or they underestimate how important it is to give people transition time once the class is over. I reinforce to these teachers in my workshops that they need to give their students plenty of time to wrap up their final relaxation time and to gather their things so that their students can maintain that 'feel good feeling' you get from a great class.

I would therefore say that the same point is true for you, when you are designing your own Genius

Break in the middle of your workday. Even if you only have 2 minutes to practice, you can take a few breaths to transition back to your workday. In these breaths, thank your mind, body and heart for embodying your practice, embrace the transition of getting back to work, and evaluate how you feel. Acknowledge to yourself that a little break really is better than no break at all.

Although this last step may seem a little self-indulgent, it has an added benefit beyond helping you to not feel so rushed. It will also help you to positively reinforce yourself for making the time to perform your Genius Break, which will in turn help support you in continuing your practice until it becomes a habit that you take for granted.

If you are lucky enough to be practicing your Genius Break with your team, friends, family members or clients, be sure to thank them for coming and to encourage them to thank themselves too.

One way to bring the centering theme that you chose into the rest of your workday, is to add the self-talk mantra you have created to your email closure or to post the message to yourself somewhere you can see it in your work station. Throughout the rest of the day, you can imagine that you are 'breathing in' this self-talk, even if you don't have time to perform a full Genius Break.

4 THE GENIUS BREAK 2/4/6//10 MOVEMENT CHECKLIST: HOW TO MAKE SURE YOU'RE MOVING EVERY MAJOR JOINT

Have you seen them?

You know, the people who walk into gyms and start randomly throwing weights around? Or the people who say they need to stretch during a meeting and start randomly moving their limbs?

I am sure these are good, decent, wonderful people.

And I suspect that they mean their body well.

But I have a sinking feeling in my stomach that they have no idea that they could be doing themselves much more harm than good.

As a kinesiologist – someone trained in the science of movement – both of these sights have made me cringe and worry for quite some time. For me, it's like watching a small child playfully run right into traffic. I want to run and scream "NO....don't do that..." when I see people moving themselves about without understanding basic biomechanics.

So here's my dilemma.

Unlike the child-care scenario, noone else can see the danger the person is putting themselves in by moving inefficiently but me (and other movement geeks like me). And, unlike a super hero, I do not wear a costume or uniform which says "Hi, I am a movement scientist...and I'd like to tell you how to stop hurting yourself." Instead, I wrote this book.

I will therefore try to boil down the wonderful and complex science of movement - kinesiology – into a very brief framework I call 2/4/6/8/10, or the mindful movement vitamin. This is by no means meant to capture all of the layers of understanding we have in kinesiology, but this will hopefully give you some important need-to-knows about how you were built structurally as a human.

What this means for you is that the movement checklist I'm about to go through with you will help you to remember that all of your joints need to move (as much as they can) every day. On some days, you will hopefully move them to the point of also getting credit for exercise and exertion. On other days, you might only move them to the degree to which you can comfortably, what we call your range of motion. Either way, this checklist can help you to make sure that you maintain your body's ability to move over time – because you will be taking the time to make sure each joint has been asked to move in the range of motions it was designed to move. As the saying goes, we must move it or lose it.

Here is my movement checklist, which was designed to make it easy for you to remember:

> 2: Move your elbows and knees in "2" directions
> 4: Move your spine in "4" directions
> 6: Move your hips in "6" directions
> 8: Move your shoulders (where your arm meets your torso) in "8" directions, and
> 10: Move the "10" digits of your hands and feet daily PLUS move "10+" minutes per day.

Please keep in mind this checklist was designed for those who do not have any medical complications with regards to the actions we are about to describe.

If you do, or if you feel any pain in any movement described next, please cease immediately. As always, you should consult your physician before beginning this or any exercise or movement regimen.

Meet The 2's:

Your Elbows and Knees (Hinge Joints)

Your arms and your legs both have joints in the middle of them called hinge joints, otherwise known as your elbows and your knees. What's important to remember about your hinge joints, is that they do have some ability to move sideways. However, if you do this too much or too quickly, they will become very upset with you (as any basketball player or tennis player will tell you).

Author's Note:

Please keep in mind that this chapter is meant to teach you basic joint actions, so that you can learn what you need to know to design your own Genius Breaks. You'll also learn my own practice for very busy days in chapter 6. As you'll find in this system, you do not have to perform the same poses or movements you see here – you can apply this system to any type of movement that you choose to do.

What this means is that although I am using yoga poses to demonstrate each joint action, you can choose to apply this same 2/4/8/10 system into any form of movement that is important for you (i.e. sports, dance, martial arts, and functional activity).

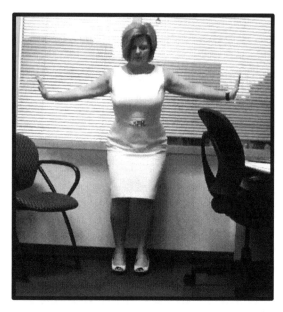

Here we see a demonstration of knee flexion (fold) and elbow extension (opening) in **Chair Pose.**

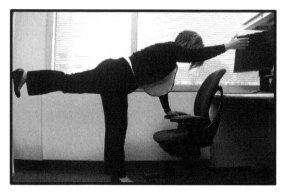

Here we see a demonstration of knee and elbow extension (open), in **Modified Warrior 3**. Please be careful if your desk chair rotates if you need balance support. The pose can also be performed with both arms in front of you or behind you (not shown).

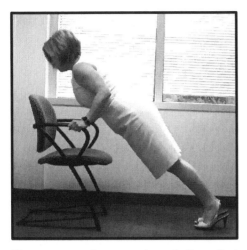

Here we see a demonstration of elbow flexion (fold) and knee extension (open), in Office Push-Ups. Here the arms are training for strength. Please DO NOT try this pose with a rolling chair.

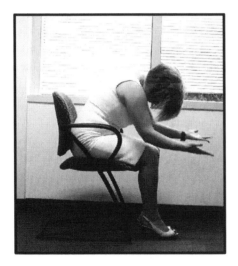

Here we see a demonstration of elbow and knee flexion, although the knees are at a 90 degree angle and the elbows are at a 45 degree angle. This pose is a great way to end your practice by releasing tension and fostering positive self-reflection.

Meet The 4's: Your Spine

Your spine is a series of compression joints; they are much like a series of hockey pucks (your vertebrae) with jelly doughnuts in between (your spongy discs). If you stepped beside yourself, and viewed yourself from the side, you would see that your spine has four major curves – at the neck (cervical), at the ribs (thoracic), at the low back (lumbar), and at your bottom (sacral). What's cool is that you can remember how many vertebrae you have in each section by remembering that you have:

Breakfast at 7 (cervical spine has 7 vertebrae)
Lunch at 12 (thoracic spine has 12 vertebrae)
Dinner at 5 (lumbar spine has 5 vertebrae)
And, depending how old you are,
You go out or go to bed at 9 (sacrum + coccyx)

Although your spine has these natural curves when you are standing tall, it usually is creating a variety of shapes throughout your day – through a combination of four primary spinal joint actions. Let's review these four actions of the spine now, so that you know how to move your spine in "4" directions daily as part of your "2/4/6/8/10" daily movement practice!

The first action is spinal flexion, which we see below:

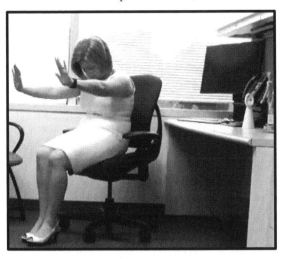

Office Seated Cat, with the spine in an active spinal flexion.

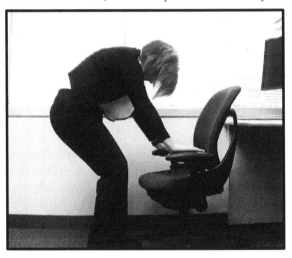

Office Standing Cat. In both poses, the abdominals are pulled in and up, and the shoulders are released away from the ears. In both poses, allow your exhale to "engage your core commitment to yourself", and to let your worries "roll off your back."

The second of our four spinal actions is a backbend, which we call spinal extension. This particular spinal movement is especially important for your workday, because it asks you to do the opposite of what your spine is most likely doing when you are seated at a desk (i.e. slouching in flexion).

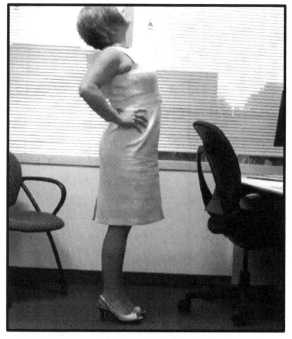

Standing Spinal Extension (Standing Camel in Yoga)

Imagine you are welcoming joy, compassion, gratitude, peace, hope, or any other positive intention into your heart. Keep your ears away from your shoulders, your neck long, and pull your shoulder blades together for an additional feeling of chest expansion and emotional fearlessness (courage in your heart).

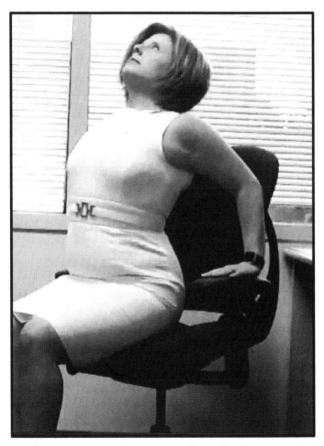

Seated Spinal Extension (Seated Camel in Yoga practice).

Both of these backbends (spinal extensions) are performed with the neck long, and the abdominals active to protect the spine. You should not feel any 'wrinkles or jagged edges' in either your neck or your low back. If you saw yourself from the side, you should look like a banana or crescent – with a smooth line from your bottom to your ears.

Remember that if you feel discomfort in these or any other pose in this book, cease immediately. You are responsible for your body, and its important to listen to its needs first and foremost.

In addition to the first two spinal joint actions of flexion and extension, you can also engage the third spinal action of spinal rotation, as shown below.

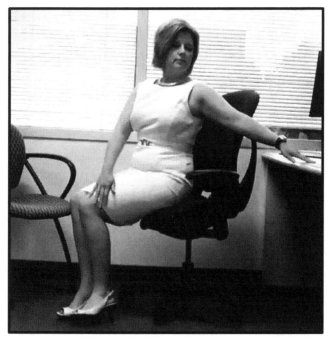

Office Twist – This is an easy spinal rotation in which you take the knees left and right, and turn your upper body in opposition to the knees. You can use the rotation capability of your desk chair to increase the range of motion – but be careful that your spine feels good while you move. Keep your spine as long as possible, since slouching makes it harder for your rotate, and keep your ears away from your shoulders.

Inhale as you sit tall on your spine, and exhale as you twist. Imagine that you are "ringing out worries" and that you are "turning to a new perspective".

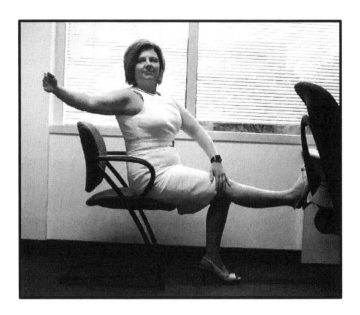

Opening Up To Opportunity -

Here you can see I am rotating the spine as in Office Twist, but I am adding two additional challenges. I am lifting the opposite leg from the direction I'm twisting to, and I am adding a bigger opening of the arm.

As with any twist, be sure to keep your spine as tall as you can so you can turn safely. When you lift one leg in front of you, you may find this difficult if the back of your legs are tight. Lift only as high as you can without slouching (and don't worry if your knee cannot fully extend to 180 degrees).

Inhale as you sit tall on your spine, and exhale as you twist. As you perform the pose, you might imagine that you are opening your heart and mind to a new direction or a new perspective.

In all forms of spinal rotation, make sure that you rotate an even number of times on each side. If you have less rotation capability on one side vs. the other, take the time to perform a few extra rotations on your weaker / less open side, so that it can "catch up" to the strength and/or flexibility level of your better side.

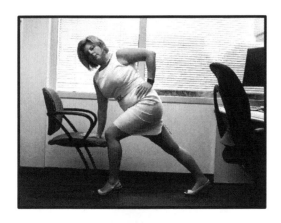

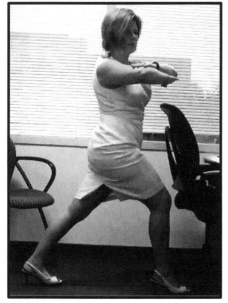

Twisting Lunge –
You can choose to hold onto the chair with your opposite arm (Top Photo), or you can see if you can perform the twist without support (Bottom Photo). Do not force any twist from the arms; allow your torso musculature to make the twist happen. Inhale to lengthen your spine; exhale to rotate so you can "turn away" from worries and doubts and "turn towards" courage and hope.

As we have seen thus far, the "4" joint actions for your spine include (1) spinal flexion, (2) spinal extension, (3) spinal rotation and now we will cover the fourth spinal action - (4) lateral flexion.

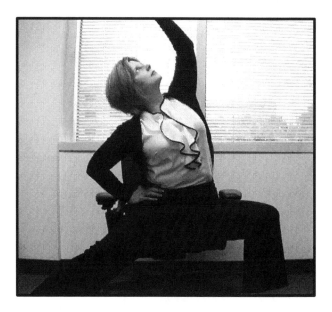

Seated Reverse Warrior from Yoga:

Here we see the spine in active lateral flexion – or side bending. Start in a seated position at the edge of your chair. Take your legs to a V Shape, with one leg in knee extension and the other in knee flexion (unless of course you are wearing a skirt) ☺.

Align yourself so that you can keep your bottom even on the chair (do not feel as though you are sitting more on your left or your right side). Allow yourself to bend sideways only as far as you can keep your bottom even on the chair. Imagine that the short side of your torso is making a little letter "c" and the long side of your torso is making a capital "C". Add or omit the arm choices shown here.

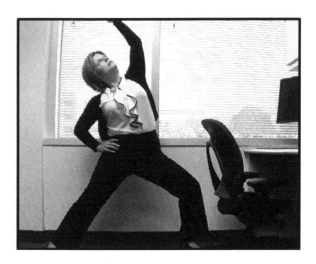

(Traditional) Reverse Warrior from Yoga:

Although many yogis consider this a basic pose, it can significantly challenge your ability to maintain your balance and your proprioception. If you are new to the pose, if you happen to be wearing heels and/or have balance issues, be especially careful that you feel steady on your legs before adding the bend.

While in the pose you can choose to bend repeatedly to each side (as though you are performing a side crunch), or to simply hold still in the pose and focus on your breath.

I suggest performing the pose along a wall (not a window or mirror) for support. Keep the hips even so that your spine receives the benefit of the stretch on your long side, and the strength-building act of engaging your internal and external obliques on your lower side.

As you allow yourself to "lean in" to your inner warrior, embrace your whole self. As you lean your body to the left and the right, engage with your left brain (embracing your inner analyst) and your right brain (embracing your inner artist). Accept that you may prefer one over the other, but that true creativity and vitality is found when we can accept the structure of our boundaries, and still creatively play within them

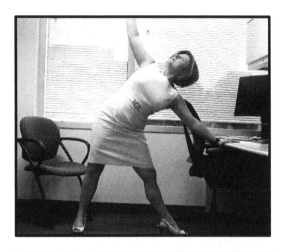

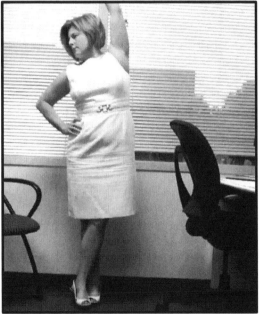

Here we see a **Gentle Triangle Pose** from Yoga (Top Photo) and **Standing Side Stretch**, inspired by Pilates Tower work (Bottom Photo). Try to bend sideways from your waist, not your neck. You can hold onto a stable surface for balance support.

These four actions of your spine [flexion, extension, rotation, and lateral flexion] enable you to do the things you need to do every day. If you have a vulnerable back (one that is in pain and/or is prone to strain, dislocation, or hypermobility) it is especially important for you to use caution with any spinal action – and to (1) avoid performing any action that is painful and (2) avoid performing any action that asks you to engage in multiple joint actions simultaneously. This is because when you perform these spinal joint actions independently one-at-a-time (as shown in the pictures above), it is safer for you. When you perform these actions simultaneously (as you do when you shovel snow or empty the dishwasher), your spine is undergoing the additional strain of compounded and sometimes contradictory torque. Listen to your body, and only move in ways your body and mind both feel good about.

Meet The 6's: Your Hips

Your hips are ball-and-socket joints, in which your femur sits nicely in your acetabulum (otherwise known as the sockets of your pelvis). Some people have a nice big open space here, while others have a more shallow space. This is why some people can easily sit in a cross legged position, and others cannot.

Unless you have a physical or medical limitation, your hips can move in six separate directions, and also make a circle – which is why we say that the hips are "six" in our 2/4/6/8/10 cheer.

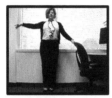

The hips can: (1) open into hip extension, as shown in the picture to the left. Yes, when you stand up you extend your hips!

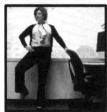

Your hips can also (2) fold into hip flexion and (3) turn out into hip external rotation as shown here. Both of these joint actions are happening here.

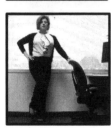

Your hips can also (2) fold into hip flexion and (4) turn in to internal rotation as shown to the left. Internal rotation is the same hip joint action you perform when you "snow plow" when you ski.

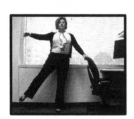

Your hips can also go sideways as shown here, as you would when you perform a jumping jack. This is called (5) abduction. And, when bring your legs back together, that is the sixth hip joint action (6) adduction.

One way that you can get your "6" actions of the hip in easily, is to perform Reverse Warrior. Yes, the same pose we saw earlier as a demonstration of lateral flexion of the spine, is also a demonstration of all six actions of the hip!

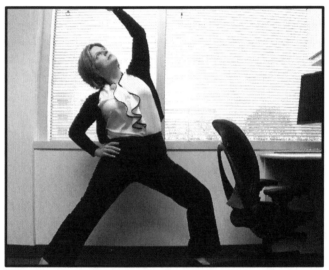

**Why Reverse Warrior Is Great For Your Hips:
Accomplish All 6 Hip Joint Actions At Once** ☺

Let's review why Reverse Warrior 2 (and the Warrior 2 Series) is great for your hips - because it asks you to perform all 6 joint actions within one pose. The bent- knee leg is in (1) hip flexion, while the opposite leg is in (2) hip extension. The bent-knee leg's hip is also turned out in (3) external rotation, while the opposite longer leg is turned into (4) internal rotation. Both legs have stepped away from the middle of the body into (5) abduction and will eventually have to come back together again through the act of hip (6) adduction. This is one of the reasons why Reverse Warrior is one of my favorite poses; it enables us to get in every action of the hip quickly and easily (and in only one pose)!

IMPORTANT:

If you have had a hip replacement or have hip pain, please do not try the moves shown above. Instead, keep the movement small and follow your doctor's guidance on appropriate range of motion.

If you have not had a hip surgery and do not otherwise have hip pain, and would like to add an additional stretch for your hips into your daily 2/4/6/8/10 practice, I find that many people I've had the pleasure of working with over the years (young and old alike) enjoy performing the following stretches. The first pose challenges your balance while extending the hip, while the other challenges your balance while externally rotating your hip.

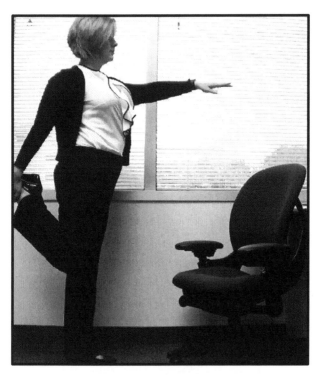

Standing Quad Stretch / Modified Dancer Pose

This pose is an example of hip extension (both legs), with an added amount of balance challenge. Please be especially careful if you have had any surgery or discomfort in the hip or the knee. Cease immediately if you have any pain or discomfort.

Secure your balance by either holding on to a stable service if necessary (not shown). Pull in on your abdominals, and take a steady exhale as you reach back and grab your back foot. Take a few breaths as you line yourself up with your knees next to each other and your spine tall. Engage your gluteals to release the hip.

As you perform the pose, you can choose to connect with a sense of groundedness (lower body), engagement (mid-body) or freedom (upper body). Measure the time on each side with breaths, rather than minutes and breathe into your past (back body), present, and future (front body).

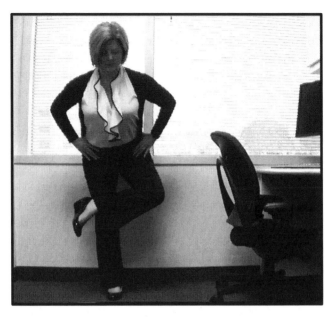

Standing Number Four / Modified Pigeon Pose

This pose is an example of hip extension (standing leg) and deep hip flexion, abduction, and external rotation (higher leg).

Secure your balance by either holding on to a stable surface if necessary (not shown), or leaning up against a wall. (Never lean on the window ☺; it is hard to tell in this picture, but I am not leaning on any surface). If the balance challenge of the pose is too intense, you can also try this pose seated.

Pull in on your abdominals, and take a steady exhale as you bring your high leg up and place your ankle above your knee.

As you breathe into the pose, imagine that you are bowing forward with a long spine made of steel – one that cannot bend.

Allow yourself to think of four things that you are grateful about your life (first side) and about your work (second pose). Breathe into the sense of gratitude you feel for both.

Now that you have learned the "2" actions (knees and elbows), the "4" actions (of the spine), the "6" action (of the hip), it is time to learn the "8" actions (of the shoulder).

Meet The 8's: Your Shoulders

Like you, your shoulders are complicated. ☺ There are actually 3 or 4 joints of the shoulder depending on which anatomy, kinesiology or physiology geek (genius) that you talk to. For our purposes we will focus on where your arm meets your torso, otherwise known as the glenohumeral joint. At this place where the arm meets the torso, you can move your arm in eight directions.

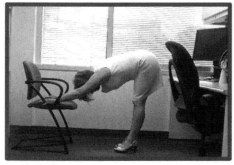

Shoulder Action 1: Flexion in Modified Downward Facing Dog

Here we see I am performing an example of the joint action of shoulder flexion. Notice it doesn't matter if you are standing up and upside down – the act of bringing your arm in front of your torso is still considered shoulder flexion.

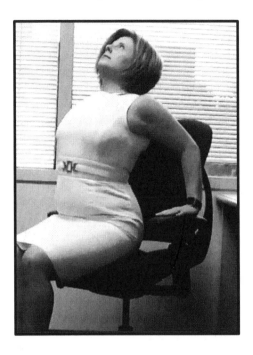

Shoulder Action 2: Extension AND
Shoulder Action 3: Internal Rotation

In the picture above, I am performing a Camel pose – which demonstrates two shoulder joint actions being performed simultaneously: (2) extension (which takes the arm behind the torso), and (3) internal rotation (which turns the upper arms downward and backwards).

It is important to note here that these two joint actions don't have to always be performed together; however, I would imagine you will find that if you take your arms into shoulder extension (behind the torso) that internal rotation feels a lot more comfortable than external rotation does.

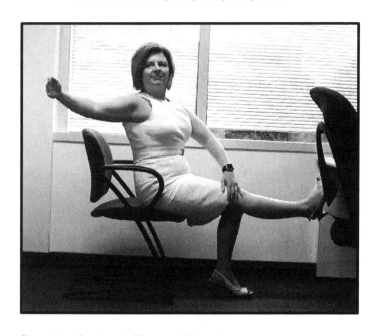

Shoulder Action 4: External Rotation,
Shoulder Action 5: Horizontal Extension AND
Shoulder Action 6: Horizontal Flexion (not shown)

Here I am (4) turning out my upper arm (External Rotation); and (5) moving my higher arm from the front of my body to the side of the room (Horizontal Extension). [If you're having a hard time visualizing what I mean, take your right arm in front of you, then take it to the side of you, parallel to the floor. That's horizontal extension – also sometimes called horizontal abduction]. Afterwards (not shown); I will move my higher arm in parallel with the floor from the side of the room, to being back in front of me. That's Horizontal Flexion, also sometimes called Horizontal Adduction].

Tip: If you go to open your arms to the sides (from the front or your torso) in order to give someone a hug you'll feel how your arms want to turn out at the shoulder, not turn in. That's because shoulder external rotation goes nicely with shoulder extension.

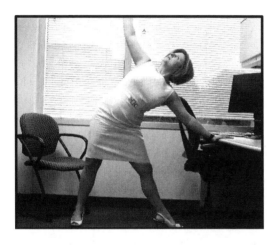

Shoulder Actions 7: Abduction AND Shoulder Action 8: Adduction

Although it is difficult to tell in the photo above, I have taken both of my arms out to the sides of the room in order to position myself into this modified triangle pose. Taking my arms to the sides of the room (in alignment with the seams of my shirt) is the act of Shoulder Abduction. Bringing them back to the seams of my dress is the act of Shoulder Adduction.

If you are having a difficult time imagining what abduction and adduction look and feel like, stand in an upright position, and then perform a jumping jack or pretend you are making an angel in the snow. The act of taking your arms to the sides of the room is abduction, and the act of bringing them back to your torso is adduction. Notice these are the same terms we use for the legs, which would be performing the same type of movement in these examples.

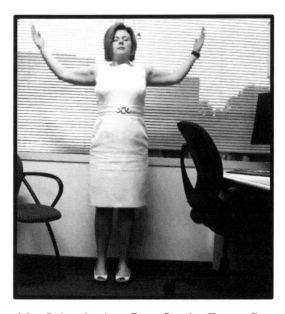

Shoulder Joint Action Case Study: Butterfly

One way to experience six out of the eight shoulder joint actions in one move is to perform a 'butterfly stroke' from swimming. As shown in the picture above you can practice the pose in your office. First you would bring you arms to the side of you (abduction), and then bring them back in front of you (flexion and internal rotation). Then you would pull you arms down into the water until they would end up behind you (extension). Then, you would rotate your shoulders outward (external rotation) so that you could take your arms out to the side (adduction, shown on page 84). The only two joint actions that would not occur directly would be horizontal extension and horizontal flexion. However, if you decided to give someone a hug after you performed your butterfly stroke, this would give you 'credit' for these last 2 joint actions for the shoulder. ☺

Meet The 10's: Your Hands and Feet

You have 10 digits in your hands and feet (fingers and toes). This "10" therefore reminds you to stretch your hands and feet, especially if they are curled up at the computer, on your smart phone and in shoes all day. Make a fist, and then make a fully extended jazz hand. If you can get away with it without upsetting your colleagues, take your shoes off and stretch your feet. I also recommend that you get two tennis balls – one for your hands and one for your feet – and that you use these to release tension in your hands and your feet as a stress and tension reliever.

Get Your "2/4/6/8/10" in every day –

When you move your body's joints in the ways that they were meant to move daily, as shown in this 2/4/6/8/10 protocol or in any way that empowers you to move in all three planes of motion, your mind, and body will benefit. Remember, that although this book demonstrates how you can plug particular yoga and office moves into the 2/4/6/8/10 system, you can analyze movement from any modality (sports, dance, etc.) from this perspective. You can also use this framework when you hit the gym. Since muscles were designed to 'move the bones around,' you'll get in a 'full body work-out' addressing 'all of your major muscle groups' if you approach your training from the 2/4/6/8/10 method.

Remember that this 2/4/6/8/10 protocol is also the framework that you can use when choosing movements to perform during your Genius Break. Research has shown that sitting for long bouts daily can either create or worsen over 26 different health conditions and that both moving and exercise are both beneficial to you – but for different reasons. In fact, some recent research has shown that exercise does not necessarily counteract the negative effects of sitting. So, moving daily (getting in your 2/4/6/8/10 requirement) AND exercising weekly are both important parts of your healthy lifestyle.

Please remember that no movement you do should feel painful, and you should always follow medical advice. If your range of motion is compromised in any joint, or if you have a condition that requires you to not move in any of the ways described here, be sure to follow medical guidance and your own body's signals so that you can heal appropriately and safely.

Now that you know your body's major joint actions, and how they move in 2/4/6/8/10 directions, its time to show you how you can add centering themes to your movement (chapter 5).

5 CENTERING SELF-TALK THEMES: THE CHAKRAS OF COMMUNICATION

"How Do You Know What to Say?"

This is actually a pretty big question for me, and I have a PhD in communication. Sometimes I don't, and sometimes I do know exactly what to say.

But here's a little secret of mine.

Whether I am designing a talk, or reacting to a moment at work, or trying to respond when someone has shared with me difficult news (for them or for me), I go to 8 centering themes, inspired by the chakras, or energy centers as they are more commonly known in Eastern medicine. Years ago I translated the chakras into centering themes, and I have refined them over the years into what I now call the Chakras of Communication.

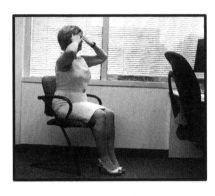

You can add a theme or two to your movement practice, or you can even focus on one theme by itself in a quiet moment as shown here.

The eight chakras of coaching themes I will review here are inspired by the following chakras:

Respect – first chakra (feet/legs)

Gratitude – second chakra (hips)

Commitment - third chakra (abs/back)

Courage - fourth chakra (heart, upper back)

Kindness –fifth chakra (mouth, ears, arms)

Insight – sixth chakra (forehead)

Community – seventh chakra (crown/top head)

Consciousness – eighth chakra (archetypes/aura)

These 8 themes are grouped into three primary communication categories (Intrapersonal,

Interpersonal and Intercultural). Under the mind-body medicine paradigm, the lower body is symbolic of our (intrapersonal) relationship with ourselves, the mid-body is symbolic of our (interpersonal) relationship with others, and the whole body is symbolic of our (intercultural) relationship with the world.

As a result, the lower body themes of respect, gratitude and commitment correspond with healing our communication with our self – intrapersonally.

The mid-body themes of commitment, courage and kindness correspond with healing our communication with our others in our life – interpersonally.

And, the upper-body themes of kindness, insight, community and consciousness correspond with healing our communication with our the world – interculturally.

You may have noticed that commitment is a theme that is connected to both the lower and the mid-body, and that kindness is a theme that is connected to both the mid-body and the upper body. That is because all of the energy centers are conceptualized as being connected and continuous. So, these two centers (commitment and kindness) are at important places of transition – from the intrapersonal to the interpersonal (commitment) and from the interpersonal to the intercultural (kindness).

Now that you know what the themes are, you may be wondering how you can choose the ones that will work best for you when you design your Genius Break.

The first bit of good news is that this is an artistic and arbitrary process – you literally cannot go wrong whether you are methodical about it or simply choose one randomly.

Allow me to share a few ways that I choose themes for my own Genius Breaks, as well as themes for the classes and workshops that I teach.

The first way that I approach choosing a centering theme (or chakra of communication) is by responding to what my body is telling me. If I have a particular area of my body that is talking to me (through pain or discomfort) I then know it would be a good idea to either (a) go to that area directly with a centering theme, or, if it is too charged or sensitive to

(b) go elsewhere to another part of my body so that I can dissipate the negative energy that may be highly focused on one particular problem (pain) area.

The second way that I choose a centering theme is to listen to what my mind is telling me. If my thoughts have key words that have embodiment hidden within them, I can literally follow the trail of clues to an area of my body and mind that may need some communicative engagement. For example, if I am having a thought that a coworker is a 'pain in my neck,' I will then focus on the kindness theme because this not only addresses the fact I am being 'mean' in my thoughts towards that person but also because I am referring to the neck area – the mind/body locality (chakra), of kindness.

The third way that I choose a centering theme for my Genius Break practice is to listen to what my heart, or feelings are telling me. Sometimes my feelings are experienced deep within my body, while others they are experienced as particular thought patterns that I can become consumed by (negative or positive). I take a step out of that 'emotional story' and decide if the conflict of this story is housed within my (1) individual (self-self conflict) experience; (2) interpersonal (self-other conflict) experience or my and (3) intercultural (self-world conflict) experience. I then choose a theme that falls under the section of the body where that conflict is found, and create a centering theme that helps me to resolve the conflict by 'retelling' and 'reclaiming' the story by both the narrative I am telling myself and the movement that I perform as gestures that help to rewrite (heal) that story.

If these processes (which are the same ones I use in my private yoga therapy practice working with clients) are not comfortable for you, you can also have fun being completely random about it (such as placing them all on notecards and then picking one randomly).

Or, you might ask yourself, and your intuition, "What part of my story do I want to focus on for today?" or "What theme feels right for me today?" Much like you just "know" which outfit you would like to wear for an important event, sometimes your intuition will help you to just "know" which centering theme will work best for your Genius Break.

If my intuition is telling me that I have to connect back with myself, I choose the themes of respect, gratitude and commitment, which are all connected to the lower body. If I need to connect more effectively with my loved ones or my coworkers, then I choose commitment, courage or kindness, because these are are all connected to the mid-body. If I need to connect more effectively in the world, I choose the theme of kindness, insight, community or consciousness, because they are housed within the upper body beyond the body.

Whatever process you use in choosing your centering theme, remember that the very act of choosing a theme and exploring which one feels right to you is in itself mindfulness at work – because the process requires that you step outside of your workday experience long enough to consider how your story is going, and what course of action you would like to take. In other words, this entire practice is a practice that fosters both engagement and stress reduction, because it asks you to step outside of your current circumstance, and to reengage with it in a way that helps you to feel as if you have the pen – so you can decide the next step of your reaction through these themes.

Once you have a centering theme (chakra of communication), you can then link it to your movement to create your Genius Break. By choosing a centering theme to add to your movement, you are not only giving yourself something to think about and say to yourself as you perform each the movement portion of your Genius Break (2/4/6/9/10), you will also transform your movement into a non-verbal gesture (of communication – a moving mantra).

Let's take a minute now to explore each centering theme, and how it is linked with the body in an embodiment perspective, in keeping with the mind/body medicine paradigm.

Respect = The Feet

This theme reminds you to respect the ground to which you stand. Your feet stand where you are, and mine stand where I am. By practicing the meaning of respect, we realize that we too have our own story, and others have theirs as well. This is symbolic of how every individual has inherent gifts, and every individual comes into any engagement with their own unique story -- with previously established patterns of thought, attitudes, behavior and values. Conflict usually occurs when we try to convince someone to see our side of reality or to "stand in our shoes" (which of course is impossible). We can persuade, and we can expose others to our perspective; however, we must respect their opinion and expect them to do the same for us in return. We can also practice the theme of respect when we honor our body's needs. We can move it more when it feels good and less when it doesn't – without competing with those who may be around us or in our heads (that we compare ourselves with). We can also think of any other behavior that does our body good as the ultimate expression of respect for ourselves.

Gratitude = The Hips

Your hips take you wherever you want to go. The hips are therefore symbolic of adaptability and change – they enable us to take a step forward, to take a step side, and to take a step back if we need to reevaluate a moment or a situation. A theme of gratitude is inspired by the hips, because it too helps us to go with the flow and adapt to the changes we find ourselves undergoing. Gratitude in the face of all things – those we wish for and those that are thrust upon us – enables us to experience joy not matter what may be occurring.

Commitment = The Torso

Your abdominals process food; your back carries your necessities and even your burdens. As a result, your torso, especially the solar plexus, is symbolic of what you choose to take in, what you choose to carry, and what you choose to let go of. When we commit fully to our selves (our beliefs, our values, our dreams, our aspirations, and our plans) we in turn are better able to commit more fully to others. And, if we find ourselves torn between commitments, we can find ourselves feeling queasy in our stomach or experiencing back pain. This center reminds you to keep that fire in your belly shining brightly – and to control its burn so that it does not go out of control nor turn too dim. By monitoring your values and your priorities, you will be able to authentically commit to yourself, your relationships and your world.

Courage = Heart Center

When we think of the heart, we think of our

deep seat of emotion and love. It is also the center for fear. Here in the heart center we always have a choice – to embrace our human fears with love. When we open ourselves up to our fears, and we allow ourselves to be vulnerable, we can then find where our true power resides. By letting go of fears (becoming more Courageous) we are better able to trust in the process of our evolution, and realize that our life and our work are practices, not perfects. At the same time, as we open our hearts we are better able to be more loving and accepting of ourselves and those we work, live and play with. Embracing the theme of courage will help you to remember that your power is within and nowhere else – and to resist the fears of doubt, regret and worry that may weigh heavy on your heart. You always have the ability and the choice to allow love to override fear.

Kindness = Mouth and Arms

Kindness is something we all agree is great to express to others, but how often do we forget to give ourselves a little kindness too? By practicing this theme, you are helping yourself to remember that if you are to truly be kind to others, it is important to start by being kind to yourself. Allow yourself to receive the nurturing, love and support of others symbolized by a wave, a kiss, and even a hug. But remember too that setting boundaries is also an act of kindness for yourself and those you love. Also, you might enjoy thinking of any health behavior as a form of kindness to your body. I have seen people think of any type of health behavior change as something that is punitive; instead of thinking of new and healthy behaviors as expressions of kindness to themselves and to those that they care about.

Insight = Forehead

To be a visionary is to be someone who can see what is possible – often before anyone else can. This is the act of placing your thoughts, beliefs, and actions in a particular line of sight, and is necessary for any personal or professional growth. By setting a goal in your future, and keeping that goal 'in sight', you increase the likelihood of that outcome becoming reality. This theme therefore reminds you to keep the big picture, and to ensure that you are keeping your internal truth in sight no matter what difficulty may be going on.

Community = Whole Body

My mother used to say that the world does not revolve around me (or any of my siblings). But the world does revolve with all of us on it – so it is important for us all to remember that we aren't here alone. That may be a simple idea, but when I see people who are successful not willing to ask for help, it makes me sad that they have forgotten that there is a whole world out there that can help them to shine. Being part of a community, at work at home or at play, really helps us to not sweat the small stuff. It also helps us to get more done in less time, since many hands make light work. Focusing on the community theme will help you to remember that you are never alone.

Consciousness = Beyond Body (Archetypes/Auras)

Some students of the chakras and practitioners of healing that use the chakra system only conceptualize seven chakras, while others believe there to be eight, twelve, or more. I personally have been trained in the understanding that there are eight, which is why I will share this eighth chakra with you.

If you think of this chakra center as connected to auras, you are buying into the idea that there is a force bigger than you and I, and that it is something that we all can tap into. In the movie Star Wars, they call it THE Force. In major religions, they call it the divine. A company calls it their mission. A family calls it their blood. A healer calls it their Source. Whatever you call it, there is something bigger and greater than each of us, beyond what the eye can actually see. When we tap into this sense of consciousness, we find a power that is beyond us and a sense of clarity that goes beyond what our eyes can see.

Another way to think of this chakra is to think of its connection to the work of Jung, and archetypes. We all have roles that we play which may or may not have anything to do with the roles that we play at work, play and home. For example, one person may have a strong mother archetype, whether or not she is a mother, because she is a nurturer at heart.

However you conceptualize it, the Consciousness centering theme (or chakra of coaching) is a theme you can go to when you want to go "beyond what the world sees" and consider your function in the world beyond the day-day roles that you or others play around you. This is where you realize a higher connection to your own story, and the lessons you are here to learn in earth school. By stepping into this theme, even if only for a few minutes, you will have the ability to connect to a bigger picture for yourself and for the problem/s you may be dealing with in front of you. You will also connect into a peace that reassures you that all is well, even if it doesn't seem to look that way in the present moment.

6 MY GO-TO GENIUS BREAK PRACTICE FOR EXTREMELY BUSY WORK DAYS

I don't like wasting time, and neither do you.

So, here goes.

This is a short-and-sweet Genius Break practice that was designed by me, for you, for your busiest days. And, true story -- I use it too.

As you will see, this practice has been designed to help you to get your sweet "2/4/6/8/10" practice in, with the least moves possible. If you are curious how we are doing that, check out the chart. The good news is that you'll get to choose your own centering communication theme to put on top of this movement. In this way, you can repeat the practice multiple times and have a unique experience every time, because you will have a different "centering lens" through which to experience it.

My Genius Break for My Busiest Days

A: Assess - Check-in with your mind, body and heart to decide if you need a calming break or an energizing break; assess the scene for safety.

B: Bones - Breathe as you move the body in 2/4/6/8/10 directions, as per chapter 3 – and as illustrated in the chart below.

C: Centering Theme - Add a chakra of communication to your movement, to operationalize mindfulness and to transform your break's movements into a gesture or "moving mantra", as per chapter 4.

E: Experience: Engage, Embrace, Embody and Evaluate (as per chapter 2).

Bones and Breath	2's	4's	6's	8's
Office Lunges with a Quad Stretch Finale	Knee Flexion (bend) and Extension (open)			
Office Chair Push-Ups	Elbow Flexion (bend) and Extension (open)			
Office Seated Cat and Cow		Spinal Flexion (cat) and Extension (cow)		
Twisting Lunge		Spinal Rotation		
Seated Reverse Warrior		Lateral Flexion (Side Bending)		
Hip Infinities with a Visit to the Barre			Takes the hips in all 6 directions	
Believe You Can Fly "Butterflies"				Takes the shoulders in all directions
Choose a Centering Theme: Respect, Gratitude, Commitment, Courage, Kindness, Insight, Community, Consciousness				
10's	Move your 10 digits (hands and toes) PLUS Move 10 minutes every day. Thank your mind, body and heart for taking a Genius Break!			

Office Lunges with a Quad Stretch Finale

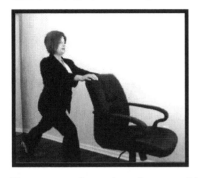 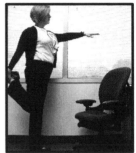

You can perform these lunges while holding onto your desk, a chair, or free-handedly. (Be careful you feel secure in your balance before letting go of any surface). While in the pose, be sure that you check to make sure your knees are not going past your toes (and that your spine is long as I am showing here. You want to practice the art of pulling in your abdominals slightly, so that you can firmly support your back. Imagine your theme is coming into your chest, and also moving freely throughout your body.

Office Chair Push-Ups

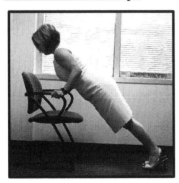

MAKE SURE YOU ARE ON A STATIONARY SURFACE - DO NOT USE A ROLLING CHAIR or MOVING SURFACE

Whether you perform your pushup with a chair, your conference table, or a nearby wall, this pose is a great way to get your body moving and to connect your mind, body and heart. If you are trying the variation at the wall, come onto your tip-toes and try to keep your body as long as you can. As you move, imagine you are literally stoking the fire of your determination with your arms. Repeat as many times as you can – without getting winded. You should be able to talk while you perform this and any move here.

Office Seated Cat

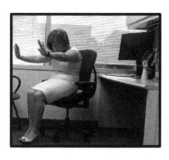

Cat pose is as an active rounding of the spine which looks a lot like a passive slump at your desk. However, it has a few important differences. First, you are pulling in and up actively on your abdominals. Second, you are actively bringing the shoulder blades away from the spine. And third you are consciously pulling in your head towards your neck, which is a great release of neck tension. In this pose, imagine that you are letting worries roll off or your back. You might even focus on the theme of kindness – as in, be kind to yourself with positive thoughts for today. You can choose to perform this pose standing if you feel the need to get out of your chair too. Repeat this pose with cow (next pose) about 4 – 10 times.

Office Seated Cow

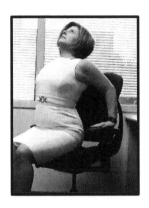

Cow pose is what we call a heart opener, which also means it is a back strengthener. Place your hands behind or underneath the shoulders, with the elbows slightly bent. Pull the shoulder blades together slightly to strengthen the back and create more breath capacity. Then, take an inhale as you lift the heart center (chest) forward and upward, without bending in the neck or low back. Keep the abdominals firm enough that the back feels supported, and loose enough that you can breathe deeply. Repeat with cat (last pose).

Lunge with a Twist

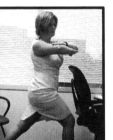

Stand tall and make sure you are secure in your feet. (You can choose to hold onto your desk or another stable surface like the wall if that helps). Take a step back behind you to a comfortable distance. Lean into your front leg, but do not allow your knee to go past your toes. Take a deep breath and exhale any tensions out of your shoulders. Inhale to grow long and tall in your spine, so that you can exhale as you turn (and pull in on your abdominals) -- imagine that you are ringing out your worries as you twist. Move on the breath – turning for every exhale and coming back to center for your inhales. Repeat both sides.

Seated Reverse Warrior

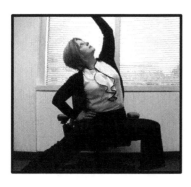

This pose is here to help you to connect with your inner warrior of peace – the part of you that is strong and steady, but not afraid to bend into the days' events and to reach up and ask for help. The pose also asks you to take your spine in a direction it doesn't always get to go – side bending, or lateral flexion. If you would like to deepen the stretch for each side of your waist, you can add a high arm. I also recommend that you keep your bottom grounded in the chair evenly – don't topple sideways like the tower of Pisa. Instead, make a nice C curve with each side of your waist. Take time to allow yourself to let your daily worries drain off to your sides. Imagine that your centering theme is above you and that you are reaching upward to it, then bringing it to your mind, and heart so you can get back to work with the warrior's peace, calm and fortitude.

Hip Infinities with a Visit to the Barre

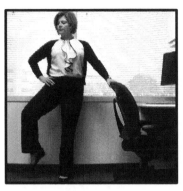

As mentioned in chapter 4, your hips move in 6 directions, and if you combine them it almost looks like you are drawing an infinity sign in front of you. (For details on how this works, please go back to chapter 2). If you are feeling adventurous (and secure) you can also try this movement with one hand holding on to a chair, or with no hands. This is a great pose to wake up your sense of balance and to help your hips to feel less tight. Plus, the act of

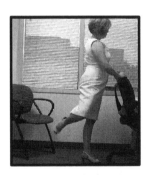

challenging your balance will reboot your mind.

If you are feeling especially feisty, you can add a few Barre-class inspired moves behind your desk chair. Start with you leg behind you and slightly bent at the knee, as shown above. Then slowly lift and lower your leg without moving your spine, and while keeping your back long. For added challenge, let go of the chair. Some might say this pose is great for getting you're a** in gear for the rest of the day ☺. These poses are great for the muscles of your gluteals, which often get weak and overstretched if you sit at an office all day.

Believe You Can Fly (Butterflies)

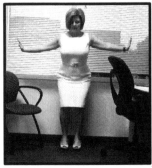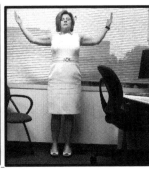

You may not necessarily believe you can fly, but in this flowing pose you can pretend like you can ☺. Imagine you are performing a butterfly stroke from swimming by taking your arms back behind you, around and up, and down in front of you. You can alternate between standing tall and bending your knees, or stand tall the whole time. Be careful that you keep your waist firm and your core tight so that the movement is mostly felt in the arms, not the back. When performed properly this flow engages every action of the glenohumeral joint (the one in which your arm meets your torso). Cease immediately if this flow is uncomfortable in any way, and open your heart to what the day has in store for you. Imagine you can literally soar over any difficulty, because you have the ability to choose how you react within your mind's eye, and your body's heart.

Back to Reality: A Mindful Minute (Choose One)

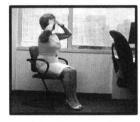 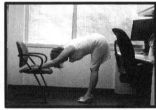

(L) **Seated Meditation** (R) **Office Downard Facing Dog**

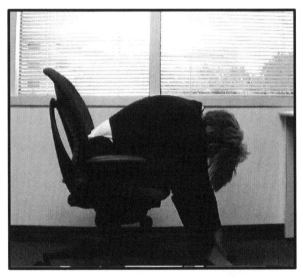

OR Child's Pose (Yoga) / Rest Position (Pilates)

It's time now to take a minute – at least -- away from everything and to focus on you before you head back to whatever your reality looks like today. Choose one of the poses shown here, depending on your preference and comfort. Now imagine your theme and enjoy giving yourself the support of that theme in your mind, your body and your heart. Thank your body and mind and heart for getting it together and stopping you from whatever busy-ness was pulling at you – so that you could take care of yourself. Take a few exhales where you release any remaining tension, and a few inhales where you imagine bringing joy, peace and equanimity to you.

Sometimes I like to add the following breath strategy:

Breathe out: Let It Go (Let It = inhale / Go = exhale).
Then I imagine that whatever is bothering me in my mind, body or heart is slowly releasing as I exhale. When I feel as though some space has been cleared (even if I don't feel completely relieved), I then turn my attention to what I do want for the day. Then, I do the following:

Breathe in: Let's Go (Let's = inhale / Go = exhale).
I then imagine that whatever outcome I desire is coming to me in its own perfect timing, including solutions to any issue or challenge I may be facing.

I take a moment to see how I feel, thank myself for practicing, and then go out into the day. I suggest you do the same – every day you can - knowing that every time you do you are fighting the effects of stress and are promoting your own body's ability to grow stronger.

And that's my go-to Genius Break practice. ☺

7 THE GEEK PART IF YOU CARE: A BRIEF WHITE PAPER ON SITTING DISEASE (SEDENTARISM)

According to the World Health Organization, approximately 3.2 million deaths each year are attributable to insufficient physical activity. (WHO, 2011). Ricciardi (2005) notes that, "research is urgently needed to describe the prevalence, risk factors, and consequences of sedentarism, and to identify the most effective intervention strategies and public policy changes to promote a physically active lifestyle".

Sitting disease (or sedentarism as it is referred to in the literature) has been referred to as the fourth highest global health risk (Sparling, et. al., 2000) that reaches across age, gender, education and socioeconomic borders (Kar, 2010). A 2011 analysis of three studies of 76 countries and over 300,000 people showed that approximately one in five people (21.4%) worldwide were considered physically inactive, or sedentary. (Dumith, Hallal, Reis, & Kohl, 2011 and Priumboom, 2011). Despite public health organization recommendations for the promotion of daily and weekly physical activity (WHO, 2010), data show that around the world, people are more sedentary; they are sitting more, and moving less.

Sedentarism can upset physical, psychological, psychosocial, mental, societal, and environmental functioning. (Bergstrom, Pisani, Tenet, Wolk, & Adami, 2001; McTiernan, 2000; Thune, 2000; Zhang, Xie, Lee, & Binns, 2004, as cited in Ricciardi, 2005; Ziemba, Chwalbinska-Moneta, Kaciuba-Uscilko, Kruk, Krzeminski, Cybulski, & Nazar, 2003, as cited in Ricciardi, 2005; Patel, Bernstein, Deka, Feigelson, Campbell, Gapstur, & Thun, 2010; Priumboom, 2011). Sedentarism has been shown to be positively correlated with a variety of adverse physiological and psychosocial health outcomes, including:

> Thermoregulation disorders, social isolation, reduction of libido, gluttony or lack of appetite, increased pain sensitivity, fatigue, concentration deficiency, attention disorders, memory problems, changes in body composition (muscle atrophy and increased fat deposits), decreased fertility, impaired hair growth and boldness, decrease of top–down decision making, self-defeating behaviour [sic] and depressive mood."
> (Priumboom, 2011)

Sedentarism has also been specifically and especially linked to cardiovascular disease. Public health researcher Steven Blair conducted a 21-year long longitudinal research study where he found that, "[M]en who reported more than 23 hours a week of sedentary activity had a 64 percent greater risk of dying from heart disease than those who reported less than 11 hours a week of sedentary activity" (Neighmond, 2011).

Defining Sedentarism

Specific and consistent definitions for sedentarism are difficult to find in the literature. However, one common trend is to distinguish between physical inactivity and sitting behavior. (Patel, Bernstein, Deka, Feigelson, Campbell, Gapstur, & Thun, 2010; Bauman, Ainsworth, Sallis, Hagströmer, Craig, Bull, & Sjöström, 2011; Ricciardi, 2005). Warren, Barry, Hooker, Sui, Church & Blair, 2010 note: "Health promotion efforts targeting physically inactive men should emphasize both reducing sedentary activity [defined as sitting behavior in this article] and increasing regular physical activity for optimal cardiovascular health" (Warren, et. al., 2010).

For simplicity, I summarize prior definitions of sedentarism found in the literature (as cited by Ricciardi, 2005) into one meta-definition. Sedentarism is defined here as (1) insufficient amounts of weekly physical activity appropriate to age level; (2) insufficient non-exercise activity (Levine, 2004); and/or (3) an undesirable surplus of daily sitting (sedentary) behavior. This new definition highlights the importance of sitting behavior as a particular and distinct aspect of sedentarism, that can be considered as a separate behavior (aspect of physical inactivity) in addition to more traditional descriptions of physical inactivity (i.e. regular weekly physical activity, and/or low levels of non-exercise activity).

Sedentary Death Syndrome:
A Slow-Moving Global Health Crisis

Sedentarism is so pervasive and related to so many adverse health outcomes, that it was termed "sedentary death syndrome" by Booth, in 2001. Interestingly, this term has unfortunately become somewhat prophetic; recent studies have confirmed sedentarism's positively correlated relationship with morbidity incidence rates. In a recent National Institutes of Health / American Association of Retired Persons diet and health study, 240,819 adults (aged 50–71 years) who did not have cancer, cardiovascular disease, or respiratory disease at baseline were examined over a 8.5 year time span. The study showed, that "time spent in sedentary behaviors was positively associated with mortality, and participation in high levels of MVPA [moderate-vigorous physical activity] did not fully mitigate health risks associated with prolonged time watching television." (Matthews, George, Moore, Bowles, Blair, Park, & Schatzkin, 2012). In other words, sitting behavior (in this case, watching television) had an adverse effect on health outcomes (disease) in populations who were otherwise physically active (engaging in MVPA's). Bauman, et. al., (2011) also notes that prolonged bouts of sitting behavior causes adverse health outcomes, that sitting time has a negative relationship with physical activity, and that time spent sitting "[W]as independently associated with total mortality, regardless of physical activity level" (Bauman, et. al, 2011).

The office worker:

Sitting in a slow-moving crisis at the office

Historically, physical inactivity was negatively associated with socioeconomic status and education level and positively associated with age (Caspersen, Pereira, & Curran 2000; Sparling & Snow 2002); however, current research indicates that physical inactivity now reaches across age, education and socioeconomic borders (Kar, 2010; Proper, et. al., 2010; Armstrong et al., 2000; Smith, et. al., 2009). Occupational sitting can lead to higher mortality outcomes (van Uffelen, 2010) and there is a positive correlation between psychosocial conditions that can affect both workplace performance and overall quality of life (namely, social isolation, fatigue, concentration deficiency, attention disorders, memory problems, decrease of top–down decision making and depressive mood. Priumboom, 2011). As a result, individuals with jobs that require extended periods of sitting are at greater risk of falling prey to the adverse health outcomes of sedentarism: physical, mental and emotional. They are at increased risk in this slow-moving global health crisis.

Sitting Disease is a Slow-Moving Crisis

According to Seeger, Sellnow & Ulmer (2011), a crisis occurs when "specific, unexpected, and non-routine events or series of events create high levels of uncertainty and threat or perceived threat to an organization's high priority goals." Using this definition of crisis, sedentarism can be considered a crisis. For individuals who must sit for extended periods during the workday, sedentarism is a crisis that is slowly posing a threat to their lives (i.e. unexpected adverse health outcomes) and also their organization's health and productivity (since ill workers are less productive and less happy).

Although the individual is generally unaware of the combined degenerative effects that prolonged sitting and/or insufficient amounts of exercise and non-exercise behavior are having on their bodies, minds, and emotions over time, they are no less at risk. As they continue through their workday at their desk chair – whether or not they stop to engage in more formal/traditional exercise – they are slowly undergoing the adverse, even deadly effects of sedentarism which take place over time.

It is especially difficult to gain a conscious understanding of a slow-moving crisis, because it is not seen readily "today." Once a crisis event (stimuli) is placed into consciousness, we can decide what to do about it (expect it, plan for it, and even create a routine for it) and how we feel about it (i.e. contextualize it as an opportunity or threat, Ulmer, Sellnow and Seeger, 2011). This transition from unconsciousness to consciousness can be caused by either the surprising and unanticipated experience of the event itself, or a discussion of the potential risk of the event. Ulmer, Sellnow and Seeger (2011) define this moment as a turning point: suggesting that the stimuli (consciousness raising moment or event) can be best seen more as an opportunity than as a threat.

In the case of a slow-moving crisis (such as sedentarism) this moment that the crisis becomes something we are conscious/aware of is especially problematic; it is sometimes not a moment at all, but a series of moments strung out over time. Since people value "today" far more than they value benefits that accrue over time (Steel & Konig, 2006) it is especially difficult for individuals to conceptualize that they are in a slow-moving crisis in the first place. And, it is also difficult to maintain the slow-moving crisis in one's everyday consciousness. These aspects of slow-moving crises make intervention design especially challenging; not only must the intervention help the individual to address the crisis, it must also create and sustain awareness and consciousness of the crisis itself over time.

Final Thoughts

Our busy lifestyles have created a world in which we move less and manage more; the rapid development of technology over the past 50 years has come with the pricetag of this dichotomy. Through the design of this movement and mindfulness public health intervention known as Genius Breaks, I hope to be part of the process of educating global citizens to the slow-moving crisis caused by our sedentary and stressful lifestyles. Ultimately, I hope to offer them global and community health solutions that do not overwhelm with fear, but instead, motivate each individual into taking crisis-solving and adaptive action – to sit less, and move more.

8 THE WOO-WOO PART IF YOU CARE: A VERY BRIEF INTRO TO WHY YOGA ISN'T ABOUT BEING PRETZEL

And it is here that I end this book with what some will find a comforting and others will find a uncomfortable thought -- the possibility that Genius Breaks can be considered a very particular form of yoga, because they meet the definition of yoga that I offer to you below.

> Yoga occurs when....
> Awareness of the physical body (in periods of movement or stillness,) is combined with positive emotional intentions and the conscious regulation of breath, in order to co-create tranquility, joy and a deeper connection to the Self, the Community and the World.

The good news is that if you do not agree that this definition accurately describes yoga, and/or you do not agree that Genius Breaks qualify as a form or style of yoga based on that definition – that is perfectly fine. Let's agree to disagree.

Or, if you would rather not consider that Genius Breaks are a form of yoga because you don't like yoga and/or that possibility scares you, that is OK Too.

I say this is all OK not only because I respect your opinion, but also because what the term "yoga" actually means is difficult to define. As an old yoga cliché states, there are many paths, but one truth.

While yogic practitioners would agree that yoga is a unique hybrid blend of science, art, global view and lifestyle, defining specific parameters around these aspects is at best, difficult. Because of this variety, one person's definition and/or understanding of yoga may not be the same as another person's. By briefly examining yoga's history, we can gain at least a panoramic view of yoga.

The word yoga is derived from the Sanskrit word "Yuj," which means to yoke, or link together. According to the Yoga Sutras of Patanjali, the ultimate aim of Yoga is to reach "Kaivalya" (emancipation or ultimate freedom of the self.) For some, this freedom is mind-based, or philosophical (i.e. freedom in the mind to enjoy a happy, balanced and blissful life.) For others, this freedom is spiritual (i.e. unification of the individual with universal oneness and divine wisdom.) Regardless of the philosophical or spiritual intentions of the practitioner, the ability to engage true self-awareness within both the mind and the body is paramount in the practice of yoga.

And, much like there are many opinions about what yoga is and isn't there are also many opinions on how one should, and shouldn't practice yoga.

Just as the arts are practiced in a variety of formats and styles (i.e. sculpting, painting, dancing, singing,) yoga is also practiced in a multitude of formats and styles. Traditionally, formats range from physical postures (asanas,) to breathwork (pranayama,) to mindfulness (including meditation and the focusing of the senses) to philosophy (theory and practices designed to create, design, and experience a life well lived and to embody spirit). Some yogis (male practitioners) and some yoginis (female practitioners) focus on one of these types of practice, while others use a combination of two or three of these.

Within each of the formats of yoga, there are also a variety of styles. Just as one musician might play a piece of music from a jazz perspective and another may play that same music from a pops perspective, the yoga formats of asanas, breathwork and mindfulness can each have their own variety of styles. For example, one person's physical poses may be very vigorous (i.e. handstands,) while another person focuses on more restorative poses (i.e. lying on the ground with a bolster under the knee.) One person's breath practice may be more invigorating, while another person's breath practice is more calming. One person's mindfulness practice may be focused on withdrawing sensory perceptions of the external environment, while another's might be focused on focusing attention into one place, situation, or creative visualization. Still others might try to freely float between thoughts, finding the space of mental stillness between them.

Although today, popular culture often considers yoga to be predominantly a physical practice, legend and oral traditions indicate that the original yogis practiced the asanas (poses and movements) in order to prepare themselves for meditation and altered states of consciousness (mindfulness and deep spirituality.) Thus, one can see the interconnectedness of the formats: the asanas, breathwork and mindfulness work well independently but also inform one another.

Suffice it to say that yoga is complex, and interpretive -- you get to decide what it is and what it isn't, and whether you are or aren't practicing it. Its beauty, its experience and its value are all found in the eye of its practitioner – not its beholder.

Which leads us back to my original thought for this chapter, and the central intention for this book. Whether or not you agree or completely disagree with me on this particular point (that Genius Breaks are a form of yoga), I hope that your Genius Breaks will enable you to experience the type of deep connection to your mind, body, heart and life that you are destined for – so that you can optimize your own unique kind of genius.

REFERENCES

Amisola, R.V., & Jacobson, M.S. (2003). Physical activity, exercise, and sedentary activity: Relationship to the causes and treatment of obesity. *Adolescent Medicine,14* (1), 23–35.

Armstrong, T., Bauman, A., & Davies, J. (2000). *Physical activity patterns of Australian adults: Results of the 1999 National Physical Activity survey.* Canberra: Australian Institute of Health and Welfare.

Barclay, E. (April 2011) Health-Chair Reform: Walk, Don't Sit At Your Desk http://www.npr.org/blogs/health/2011/04/28/135766887/health-chair-reform-walk-dont-sit-at-your-desk.

Bauman, A., Ainsworth, B. E., Sallis, J. F., Hagströmer, M., Craig, C. L., Bull, F. C., and Sjöström, M. (2011). The Descriptive Epidemiology of Sitting: A 20-Country Comparison Using the International Physical Activity Questionnaire (IPAQ). *American Journal Of Preventive Medicine, 41*(2), 228-235.

Bergstrom, A.; Pisani, A.; Tenet, V.; Wolk, A.; & Adami, H. O. (2001). Overweight as an avoidable cause of cancer in Europe. *International Journal of Cancer, 91,* 421–430 as cited in Ricciardi, R. (2005). Sedentarism: a concept analysis. *Nursing Forum, 40*(3), 79-87.

Bernstein, M. (1999). Definition and Prevalence of Sedentarism in an Urban Population. American Journal Of Public Health, 89(6), 862 as cited in Ricciardi, R. (2005). Sedentarism: a concept analysis. *Nursing Forum, 40*(3), 81.

Block, L. G., & Punam, K. A. (1995). When to Accentuate the Negative: The effectsof perceived efficacy and message framing on intentions to perform a health-related behaviour. *Journal of Marketing Research 32* (2): 192- 204.

Booth, F. W. (2001) Researchers Against Inactivity Disorders. Retrieved December 1, 2011 from http://hac.missouri.edu/rid/

Booth, F. W., et al. (2002). Waging war on physical inactivity: Using modern molecular ammunition against an ancient enemy. *Journal of Applied Physiology (93)*:3-30; as cited in Sparling, P. (2003). College physical education: An unrecognized agent of change in combating inactivity-related diseases. *Perspectives in Biology and Medicine, 46*(4), 579-87.

Brooks, F., & Magnusson, J. (2006). Taking Part Counts: Adolescents' Experiences of the Transition from Inactivity to Active Participation in School-Based Physical Education. *Health Education Research, 21*(6), 872.

Carmack, S. (2014). *Making Sense of Well-Being: Mixed-method study applying sense-making theory to explore the role of communication competence and social support in physical, emotional, mental and comprehensive well-being.* (Doctoral Dissertaiton). George Mason University. http://digilib.gmu.edu.

Carmack, S. (2015). *Well-Being Ultimatum: A Self-Care Guide for Strategic Healers.* Body Doctrine Press: Fairfax, VA.

Carmody, J., & Baer, R. A. (2008). Relationships between mindfulness practice and levels of mindfulness, medical and psychological symptoms and well-being in a mindfulness-based stress reduction program. *Journal Of Behavioral Medicine, 31*(1), 23-33.

Caspersen, C. J., M. A. Pereira, and K. M. Curran. 2000. Changes in physical activity patterns in the United States, by sex and cross-sectional age. *Medical Science Sports and Exercise 32*: 1601-9; as cited in Sparling, P. B. (2003). College physical education: An unrecognized agent of change in combating inactivity-related diseases. *Perspectives in Biology and Medicine, 46*(4), 579-87.

Deitz, W.H. (1996). The role of lifestyle in health: The epidemiology and consequences of inactivity. *Proceedings of the Nutrition Society, 55*, 829–840 as cited in Ricciardi, R. (2005). Sedentarism: a concept analysis. *Nursing Forum, 40*(3), 79-87.

Dumith, S. C., Hallal, P. C., Reis, R. S., & Kohl, H. W. (2011). Worldwide prevalence of physical inactivity and its association with human development index in 76 countries. Preventive Medicine, 53(1/2), 24-28.

Fishbein, M., & Ajzen, I. (2010). *Predicting and changing behavior: The reasoned action approach.* New York: Psychology Press.

Frazer, C. F., Sheehan, K. B., & Charles, P.H. (2002). Patti Charles H. Advertising strategy andeffective advertising: comparing the USA and Australia. *Journal of MarketingCommunications 8* (3, September): 149-164.

Gardiner, P. A., Healy, G. N., Eakin, E. G., Clark, B. K., Dunstan, D. W., Shaw, J. E., and Owen, N. (2011). Associations Between Television Viewing Time and Overall Sitting Time with the Metabolic Syndrome in Older Men and Women: The Australian Diabetes Obesity and Lifestyle

Study. *Journal Of The American Geriatrics Society*, *59*(5), 788-796.

Gilson, N. D., Puig-Ribera, A. A., McKenna, J. J., Brown, W. J., Burton, N. W., & Cooke, C. B. (2009). Do walking strategies to increase physical activity reduce reported sitting in workplaces: a randomized control trial. *International Journal Of Behavioral Nutrition And Physical Activity*, *6*(43), (20 July 2009).

Homer, P. M., & Yoon, S. (1992). Message framing and the interrelationships among ad-based feelings, affect, and cognition. *Journal of Advertising 21* (1) pp19-34.

Kar, S., Thakur, J., Virdi, N., Jain, S., & Kumar, R. (2010). Risk factors for cardiovascular diseases: is the social gradient reversing in northern India?. *The National Medical Journal Of India*, *23*(4), 206-209.

Katzmarzyk, P. T. (2004). Perspective: sedentary death syndrome - where to from here?. *Canadian Journal Of Applied Physiology*, *29*(4), 444-446.

Levine, J. (2004). Non-exercise activity thermogenesis (NEAT). *Nutrition Reviews*, *62*(7 Pt 2),S82-S97.

Matthews, C., George, S., Moore, S., Bowles, H., Blair, A., Park, Y., & ... Schatzkin, A. (2012). Amount of time spent in sedentary behaviors and cause-specific mortality in US adults. *American Journal Of Clinical Nutrition*, *95*(2), 437-445. doi:10.3945/ajcn.111.019620

McTiernan, A. (2000). Associations between energy balance and body mass index and risk of breast carcinoma in women from diverse racial and ethnic backgrounds in the U.S. *Cancer, 88*,1248–1255 as cited in Ricciardi, R. (2005). Sedentarism: a concept analysis. *Nursing Forum, 40*(3), 79-87.

Neighmond, P. (2011) Sitting All Day: Worse for You Than You Might Think. www.npr.org. http://www.npr.org/2011/04/25/135575490/sitting-all-day-worse-for-you-than-you-might-think.

Nelson, K.M., Reiber, G., & Boyko, E.J. (2002). Diet and exercise among adults with type 2 diabetes: Findings from the third national health and nutrition examination survey (NHANES III). Diabetes Care, 25 (10), 1722–1728.as cited in Ricciardi, R. (2005). Sedentarism: a concept analysis. *Nursing Forum, 40*(3), 79-87.

Patel, A. V., Bernstein, L., Deka, A., Feigelson, H., Campbell, P. T.,

Gapstur, S. M., and Thun, M. J. (2010). Leisure Time Spent Sitting in Relation to Total Mortality in a Prospective Cohort of US Adults. *American Journal Of Epidemiology*, *172*(4), 419-429.

Patten, S.B.; Williams, J.V.; Lavorato, D.H.; and Eliasziw, M. (2009) A longitudinal community study of major depression and physical activity. *General Hospital Psychiatry 31*:571–575.

Posadzki, P., & Parekh, S. (2009). Yoga and physiotherapy: A speculative review and conceptual synthesis. Chinese Journal of Integrative Medicine, 15, 66-72.

Proper, K. I., Cerin, E. E., Brown, W. J., & Owen, N. N. (2007). Sitting time and socio-economic differences in overweight and obesity. *International Journal Of Obesity*, *31*(1), 169-176.

Pullman, A. W., Masters, R. C., Zalot, L. C., Carde, L. E., Saraiva, M. M., Dam, Y., & ... Duncan, A. M. (2009). Effect of the transition from high school to university on anthropometric and lifestyle variables in males. *Applied Physiology, Nutrition & Metabolism*, *34*(2), 162-171. doi:10.1139/H09-007

Pruimboom, L. (2011). Physical inactivity is a disease synonymous for a non-permissive brain disorder *Medical Hypotheses 77* (5) 708–713

Ricciardi, R. (2005). Sedentarism: a concept analysis. *Nursing Forum, 40*(3), 79-87.

Schoormans, D., & Nyklíček, I. (2011). Mindfulness and Psychologic Well-Being: Are They Related to Type of Meditation Technique Practiced?. *Journal Of Alternative & Complementary Medicine*, *17*(7), 629-634.

Seligman, M. (2004). Foreword. In P. Linley & S. Joseph (Eds.), Positive psychology in practice (pp. xi-xiii). Hoboken, NJ: John Wiley and Sons.

Smith, M., Chen, C. M., & McKyer, E. J. (2009). University Faculty Modeling Health Promoting Behaviors: Meeting surgeon general's guidelines for physical activity. *American Journal Of Health Studies*, *24*(4), 380-385.

Sparling, P. B., et al. 2000. Promoting physical activity: The new imperative for public health. Health Educ. Res. 15:367-76; as cited in Phillip B Sparling. (2003). College physical education: An unrecognized agent of change in combating inactivity-related diseases. Perspectives in Biology and Medicine, 46(4), 579-87.

Sparling, P. B., and T. K. Snow. 2002. Physical activity patterns in recent college alumni. *Research Quarterly in Exercise and Sport, 73.* 200-205; as cited in Sparling, P.B. (2003). College physical education: An unrecognized agent of change in combating inactivity-related diseases. *Perspectives in Biology and Medicine, 46*(4), 579-87.

Speakman, J.R. (2004). Obesity: The integrated roles of environment and genetics. Journal of *Nutrition, 134 (8S),* 2090–2105 as cited in Ricciardi, R. (2005). Sedentarism: a concept analysis. Nursing Forum, 40(3), 79-87.

Thesenvitz, J. (2000). *Understanding and using fear appeals for tobacco control.* Toronto, Ontario, Canada: Council for a Tobacco-Free Ontario, The Program Training and Consultation Centre and The Health Communication Unit (University of Toronto).

Thune, I. (2000). Assessments of physical activity and cancer risk. European Journal of *Cancer Prevention, 9,* 387–393 as cited in Ricciardi, R. (2005). Sedentarism: a concept analysis. *Nursing Forum, 40*(3), 79-87.

Tudor-Locke, C.E., & Myers, A.M. (2001). Challenges and opportunities for measuring physical activities in adults. *Sports Medicine, 31* (2), 91–100 as cited in Ricciardi, R. (2005). Sedentarism: a concept analysis. *Nursing Forum, 40*(3), 79-87.

Uffelen, J., Watson, M., Dobson, A., & Brown, W. (2011). Comparison of Self-Reported Week-Day and Weekend-Day Sitting Time and Weekly Time-Use: Results from the Australian Longitudinal Study on Women's Health. *International Journal Of Behavioral Medicine, 18*(3), 221-228.

van Uffelen, J. Z., Wong, J., Chau, J. Y., van der Ploeg, H. P., Riphagen, I., Gilson, N. D., & Brown, W. J. (2010). Occupational Sitting and Health Risks: A Systematic Review. *American Journal Of Preventive Medicine, 39*(4), 379-388. doi:10.1016/j.amepre.2010.05.024
Warren, T. Y.; Barry, V.; Hooker, S.P.; Sui, X.; Church, T.S.; Blair, S.N. (2010). Sedentary Behaviors Increase Risk of Cardiovascular Disease Mortality in Men. *Medicine, Sport and Exercise (42)* 5:879-885.

Wheatley, J. J. & Sadaomi, O. (1970) The relationship between anxiety and positive and negative advertising appeals. *Journal of Marketing Research* (7) 85-89.

Witte, K. & Roberto, A. J. (in press). Fear appeals and public health: Managing fear and creating hope. In L. Frey and K. N. Cissna (Eds.), *Handbook of applied communication.* Fort Worth, TX: Harcourt Brace

Jovanovich.

Witte, K. (1992). Putting the fear back into fear appeals: The extended parallel process model. *Communication Monographs, 59*, 329-349.

World Health Organization (WHO) (2011). Physical Inactivity: A Global Public Health Problem. December 2011 from: http://www.who.int/dietphysicalactivity/factsheet_inactivity/ en/index.html.

Zhang, M., Xie, X., Lee, A.H., & Binns, C.W. (2004). Sedentary behaviors and epithelial ovarian cancer risk. *Cancer Causes and Control,15*, 83–89 as cited in Ricciardi, R. (2005). Sedentarism: a concept analysis. *Nursing Forum, 40*(3), 79-87.

Ziemba, A.W., Chwalbinska-Moneta, J., Kaciuba-Uscilko, H., Kruk, B., Krzeminski, K., Cybulski, G., & Nazar, K. (2003). Early effects of short-term aerobic training. Physiological responses to graded exercise. *Journal of Sports Medicine and Physical Fitness, 43* (1), 57–63 as cited in Ricciardi, R. (2005). Sedentarism: a concept analysis. *Nursing Forum, 40*(3), 79-87.

ABOUT THE AUTHOR

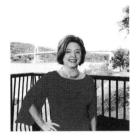

Dr. Suzie Carmack is an interdisciplinary scholar, strategist, speaker, and survivor who has been promoting health, wellness and well-being since 1997. As a pioneer in the fields of integrative health coaching, movement therapy and well-being promotion, she has extensive experience as a thought-leader, executive coach, university professor, and yoga teacher and coach trainer. She is the author of <u>Well-Being Ultimatum (2015)</u> and has presented her unique approach to moving people mindfully during their work or school day in over 100 keynotes and conference presentations worldwide. Her workplace move-at-your-desk and mindful leadership programs have inspired over 30,000 people from 89 countries to move mindfully during their workday, and in so doing, to fight the public health and biopsychosocial well-being risks of work/life stress and sitting disease (sedentarism). As a private integrative health coach and mindful movement therapist, she has personally coached over 1000 C-suite executives, clinicians, educators, and senior-ranking military officers in the art and science of moving and living well. As an interdisciplinary scholar, she holds advanced degrees in the social sciences (PhD, Health Communication), natural sciences (MEd, Kinesiology) and Humanities (MFA, Theatre), as well as multiple practitioner credentials in the science of movement (PMA-CPT, ERYT, and ACE-CPT). She lives with her partner Bob and her daughter Sophia and is also the mother of two amazing young men: Chris, and Brandon. Learn more about how you can join Dr. Carmack and help move the world to sit less and move more in the Genius Break Community at **www.DrSuzieCarmack.com.**

Dr. Suzie Carmack, PhD, MFA, MEd, ERYT

Thank you for reading.
Thank you for moving.
Thank you for sharing.
And remember…

Be Yourself. Everyone else is already taken
– Oscar Wilde

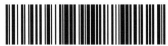
Made in the USA
Middletown, DE
22 February 2019